△△△△△△△△△△△△△△△△△△△△△△△△△△△△△△△△△△△△△

Diabetes
Meal
Planning
Made
Easy

How to Put the Food Pyramid to Work
for Your Busy Lifestyle

Hope S. Warshaw, MMSc, RD, CDE

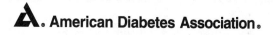

American Diabetes Association.

△△△△△△△△△△△△△△△△△△△△△△△△△△△△△△△△△△△△△

Publisher   Susan H. Lau
Editorial Director   Peter Banks
Production Director   Carolyn Segree
Editor and Designer   Sherrye Landrum
Illustrations   Rebecca Grace Jones
Cover Design   Wickham & Associates
Reviewers   Patti Bazel Geil, MS, RD,CDE,
Phyllis Barrier, MS, RD, CDE, Janine Freeman, RD, CDE, and
Carolyn Leontos, RD, CDE, MS,

American Diabetes Association
1660 Duke Street
Alexandria, VA 22314

Library of Congress Cataloging-in-Publication Data

Warshaw, Hope, 1954–
  Diabetes meal planning made easy: how to put the food pyramid to work
  for your busy lifestyle/Hope Warshaw.

      p.   cm.
  Includes index.
  ISBN 0-945448-61-9
  1. Diabetes--diet therapy. I. Title.
RC662.W315   1996
616.4'620654--dc20

                                                                96-18948
                                                                CIP

Printed in the United States of America

3 5 7 9 10 8 6 4

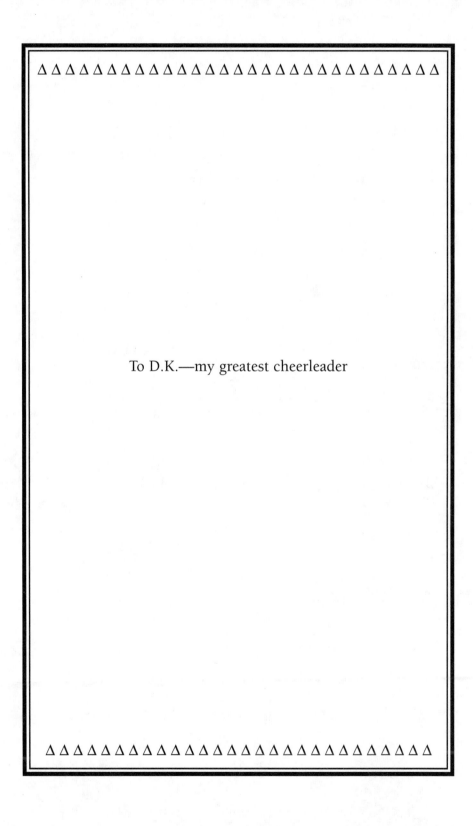

To D.K.—my greatest cheerleader

△ △

CONTENTS

△ △

△ △

△ △

△ △

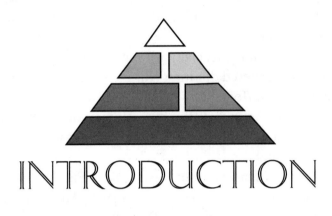

INTRODUCTION

Most people agree that meal planning is the most difficult part of managing diabetes. That's understandable. It is hard work to eat certain foods in measured amounts and at regular times—every day, 365 days a year. That just doesn't fit well with today's fast-paced lifestyle. This book is designed to give you a hand with this daily challenge.

The food you eat makes your blood glucose rise. In fact, what you eat affects your blood glucose, cholesterol, blood pressure, weight, and long-term complications. That's why this book was written.

Meal planning is one of the three parts of the diabetes "balancing act" or triangle. The others are physical activity and diabetes medications (for some people). When you check your blood glucose daily, you have feedback to let you know whether you are in or out of balance. With records of these daily checks, you and your health-care provider can make changes, if needed, to your meal plan, your medication, or your physical activity to get your blood glucose levels closer to normal.

A meal plan tells you how many carbohydrates, proteins, fats, vitamins, and minerals you need and how many servings from each

1

food group you should eat at different meals and snacks. Your meal plan should be based on your food preferences, usual schedule, and lifestyle. It is not a rigid set of numbers but ought to be flexible enough to cover every situation from a special occasion to a sick day. And don't worry, you don't have to leave all your favorite foods and recipes behind.

To learn about and succeed with meal planning, you will need to work with a registered dietitian (RD) who has experience in diabetes management. Together you will find the best way to plan meals and snacks. Your dietitian can help you make small changes in your eating habits and work toward your long-term goals of diabetes management.

Diabetes Meal Planning Made Easy: How to Put the Food Pyramid to Work for Your Busy Lifestyle uses the American Diabetes Association and The American Dietetic Association's Diabetes Food Pyramid to teach you an easy way to make healthy food choices and put healthy meals and snacks together. Every food fits into the food pyramid. We know that you have little time to plan, shop for, and cook healthy meals. That's why *Diabetes Meal Planning Made Easy* offers you quick and easy ways to eat more fruits and vegetables, trim your fat grams, make realistic changes in your eating habits, use Nutrition Facts on the food label, and enjoy eating out. Each chapter offers you new ways to use a meal plan to simplify your daily life.

The nutrition information in this book is in part from the American Diabetes Association and The American Dietetic Association's *Exchange Lists for Meal Planning* nutrient database. In addition, nutrition information is from several other sources, including Nutrition Facts from food labels; N-Squared Nutrition Analysis, First Data Bank, San Bruno, California; and NutriBase, Phoenix, Arizona.

△△△△△△△△△△△△△△△△△△△△△△△△△△△△△△△△△△

PART ONE

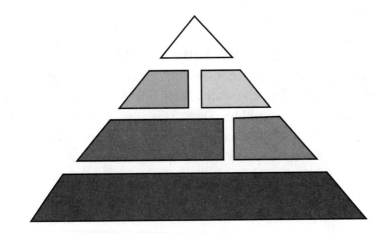

△△△△△△△△△△△△△△△△△△△△△△△△△△△△△△△△△△

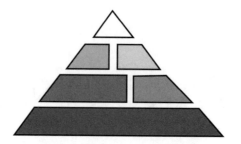

CHAPTER 1

THE NEW GUIDELINES FOR HEALTHFUL EATING

Over the last 40 years, the American Diabetes Association has revised its guidelines for healthy eating several times—most recently in 1994. These new recommendations challenge a number of long-held beliefs about diabetes and nutrition. This chapter explains the 1994 nutrition recommendations.

Eat healthfully together

The diabetes nutrition recommendations are the same as the *Dietary Guidelines for Americans* from the Department of Health and Human Services and U.S. Department of Agriculture (USDA). You don't need to buy special foods or prepare special meals. The USDA Food Guide Pyramid shows you how these suggestions become the foods you choose. The whole family follows the same healthy eating guidelines:

▲ Eat a variety of food.

▲ Balance the food you eat with physical activity—to maintain or improve your weight.

▲ Choose a diet with plenty of grain products, vegetables, and fruits.

▲ Choose a diet low in fat, saturated fat, and cholesterol.

4

▲ Choose a diet moderate in sugars.

▲ Choose a diet moderate in salt and sodium.

▲ If you drink alcoholic beverages, do so in moderation.

What to eat when you have diabetes

Protein

Only about 10–20% of your calories should come from protein. Protein is found mainly in meats, poultry, seafood, and dairy foods. Starches, vegetables, and fruits also contain small amounts of protein. Unfortunately, most Americans eat more animal protein (for example, meats and dairy foods) than nonanimal protein (for example, grains and vegetables). People with diabetes don't need any more or any less protein than the general public.

Fat and carbohydrate

If 10–20% of your calories come from protein, then you can divide the remaining 80–90% between the two other main sources of calories—fat and carbohydrate. In general, 20–40% of calories might come from fat and 40–50% from carbohydrate.

Fat

Fat is divided by structure into three types: saturated, polyunsaturated, and monounsaturated. Examples of the three types are

▲ Saturated—meats and whole milk dairy foods

▲ Polyunsaturated—corn or soybean oil

▲ Monounsaturated—canola or olive oil

The guidelines strongly recommend keeping saturated fat to less than 10% of your calories. That means limiting animal protein and whole milk dairy foods. Likewise, try to keep polyunsaturated fat to less than 10% of your calories. Monounsaturated fats, however, might help lower blood cholesterol and raise the good cholesterol—high-density lipoproteins (HDL). That's why we recommend that you get at least 10% of your fat from monounsaturated fats, such as canola and olive oil. (See chapter 8.)

Carbohydrates—Starches and Sugars

Starches such as pasta, potatoes, and cereals are among the healthiest foods you can eat. We include sugars with starches because they are carbohydrates too. Sugars do not raise blood glucose any faster than do starches. That is startling news for people with diabetes. The 1994 nutrition recommendations say that it is more important to eat the same amount of carbohydrate at the same meal day after day than to worry about whether the carbohydrate comes from starches or sugars. All carbohydrates raise blood glucose about the same. Whether you eat 15 g of carbohydrate from seven Lifesavers or 15 g of carbohydrate from 1/2 cup of pasta, your blood glucose rise will be about the same.

Other things affect how quickly different carbohydrates raise your blood glucose: whether the food is raw or cooked, your portion size, how much protein and fat are in the meal, how quickly you eat, what your blood glucose is at the time of the meal, and how much and what type of insulin or diabetes pills are in your body.

Sugars and sweets

The guideline for sugars and sweets is not the OK for a sugar free-for-all. Yes, you can include your favorite dessert in your meal plan from time to time. But too many sugars and sweets are unhealthy for anyone. They are high in calories but low in nutrients. Plus, sweets, such as cheesecake and regular ice cream, are high in fat too. Find out from your RD how many servings of sugars and sweets are OK for you based on your weight, blood glucose control, and diabetes goals. Remember, eat sugar in moderation.

Dietary fiber

Examples of foods with fiber are whole wheat bread, bran cereal, peas, and lentils. The recommendation for everyone is 20–35 g of fiber each day. The problem is that most Americans eat only about 10–13 g each day. You can get about 5 g of dietary fiber from a serving of a whole-grain cereal, a third of a cantaloupe, or 1/2 cup of cooked lentils. Your digestion works better and you are healthier when you include fiber in your diet.

Sodium

The recommendation for sodium is between 2400 and 3000 mg per day. Most Americans consume an average of 4000–6000 mg per day. For people with high blood pressure, the recommendation is 2400 mg or less per day. To help you picture how much that is, 1/4 teaspoon of salt has 450 mg of sodium, 1 oz processed American cheese has 400 mg, and 8 oz of milk has 120 mg.

Alcohol

No more than 1–2 drinks a day should be consumed. For everyone, with or without diabetes, drinking too much alcohol can be both a health and a safety hazard. Alcohol adds many calories—1 1/2 oz (a jigger) of whiskey or vodka contains 100 calories but few nutrients. It can raise triglycerides and is the cause of many car accidents. For people with diabetes taking insulin or diabetes pills, alcohol often lowers blood glucose, sometimes dangerously so.

Vitamins and minerals

If you are eating a variety of foods chosen mostly from the bottom two levels of the pyramid and your blood glucose is controlled, you probably don't need vitamin and mineral supplements. Your health-care team may recommend supplements if you have difficulty getting all you need from foods, for instance, if you are a strict vegetarian, are on a weight-reducing meal plan that is 1200 calories or less per day, are pregnant or breastfeeding, or have certain short- or long-term illnesses. Ask your health-care team any questions you may have about vitamin and mineral supplements.

Reasons for the new recommendations

No "diabetic diet"

You might have been given a diet on a pre-printed sheet for a calorie level—1200, 1500, and so on. But there is no such thing as a "diabetic diet." People with diabetes follow the same healthy eating guidelines that all Americans do. You don't need any special foods. An RD can help you design a meal plan based on your nutrition needs and your lifestyle. For instance, the meal plan for a vegetarian who works an evening shift will be different from the meal plan of someone who lives alone and eats 90% of meals in restaurants.

More than one meal-planning approach

The American Diabetes Association and The American Dietetic Association have developed several ways to plan meals: the *Exchange Lists for Meal Planning,* Carbohydrate Counting Levels 1–3, and the *First Step in Meal Planning* based on the Diabetes Food Pyramid. This book shows you how to use the Diabetes Food Pyramid.

Individualization is key

You need to work with a dietitian to develop a meal plan just for you. You should consider all of your health, diabetes, and nutrition goals. Also consider your food preferences; when you like to eat; whether you like or need snacks at certain times; your schedule, including weekdays and weekends; types of exercise you do and your physical activity schedule; and, most important, what you want to do.

It is common for people with diabetes, especially type II diabetes, to have high blood cholesterol, high low-density lipoprotein (LDL), low HDL, high triglycerides, and high blood pressure. Any changes you make to your meal plan for diabetes-related conditions will also help prevent diseases such as heart disease, high blood pressure, and diabetes.

You need flexibility

In our fast-paced world, life doesn't always go according to plan. Your meal plan needs to be flexible enough that you can delay a meal or snack or eat at a restaurant or use convenience foods. It must stretch to fit the days when your activity level is way up— perhaps a weekend hike or day of skiing—and the days when you feel ill and have no appetite. You can learn how to manage these situations from your diabetes educators.

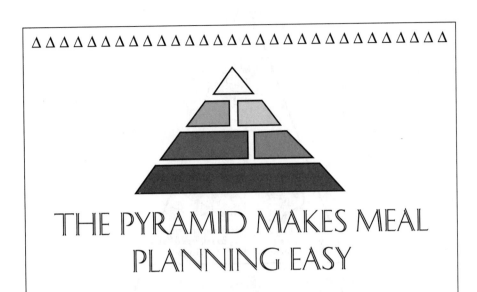

CHAPTER 2

THE PYRAMID MAKES MEAL PLANNING EASY

Why a pyramid?

A pyramid is easy to remember. When you hear the word you get a clear picture of a triangle in your mind. The large sections at the bottom are the foods you should eat more of, and you should eat less of the foods that occupy the small space at the top.

Diabetes gets its own food pyramid

In 1995, the American Diabetes Association and The American Dietetic Association adapted the USDA Food Guide Pyramid in a pamphlet called *The First Step in Diabetes Meal Planning*. The Diabetes Food Pyramid translates the healthy eating concepts in the USDA Food Guide Pyramid for diabetes meal planning. There are only a few differences—in the fine print. Compare the two pyramids on the next pages to see. Each has five main food groups, but the names of the food groups are slightly different.

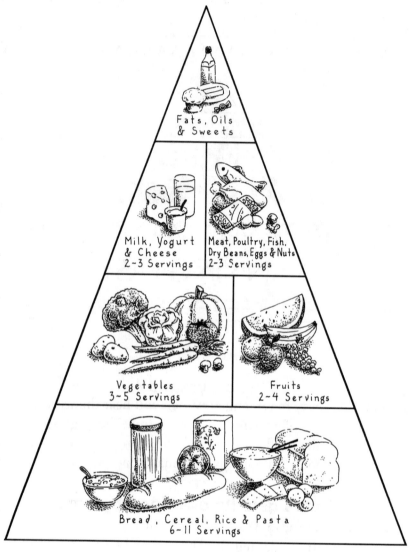

USDA FOOD GUIDE PYRAMID

The name of the food group at the tip of the pyramid is different: some foods are listed in different groups. In the Diabetes Pyramid, beans are in the starch group and cheese is in the meat group. In the USDA pyramid, beans are in the meat group and cheese is in the milk group.

In the USDA pyramid, alcohol is not mentioned. In the diabetes pyramid, alcohol is included in the group at the top, along with fats and sweets. Both pyramids encourage limiting these items.

The USDA Food Guide Pyramid is used on food labels, on information pamphlets from food companies, and on government nutrition education materials. You can use both pyramids to remind you what foods to eat each day.

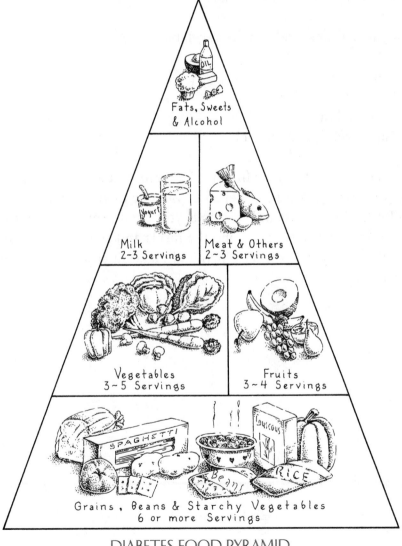

DIABETES FOOD PYRAMID

How to work the diabetes pyramid

The diabetes pyramid has six sections for food groups. They vary in size. The largest group—grains, beans, and starchy vegetables—is on the bottom. This means that you should eat more servings of grains, beans, and starchy vegetables than of any of the other foods. The smallest group—fats, sweets, and alcohol—is at the top of the pyramid; this tells you to eat very few servings. These are the six food groups, from the base up:

1. Grains, beans, and starchy vegetables
2. Vegetables
3. Fruits
4. Milk
5. Meat and others
6. Fats, sweets, and alcohol

Eat servings from the first five food groups every day. The number of servings you need depends on your diabetes goals, calorie and nutrition needs, and the foods you like to eat. You can divide the number of servings among the meals and snacks you're going to eat that day. The diabetes pyramid makes it easier to remember what to eat.

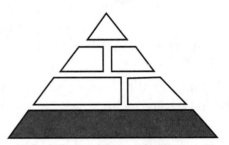

CHAPTER 3

THE BASE—GRAINS, BEANS, AND STARCHY VEGETABLES

What you will learn

▲ Everyone, including people with diabetes, should eat more starches.

▲ How starches get into fat trouble.

▲ The number of servings of grains, beans, and starchy vegetables to eat each day.

▲ Serving sizes of grains, beans, and starchy vegetables.

▲ Easy ways to eat more grains, beans, and starchy vegetables.

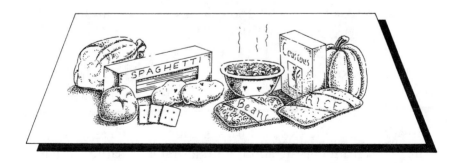

Form a firm foundation

Grains, beans, and starchy vegetables—starches—are the base of the pyramid, the largest space. The pyramid is telling you to make grains, beans, and starchy vegetables the foundation of all your meals and snacks. Starches should be the first foods you choose. Build meals and snacks around grains, beans, and starchy vegetables, such as pasta topped with tomato and mushroom sauce, bean burritos, or couscous covered with vegetable and lamb stew.

America's report card on starches

We have done it backward for years. Meat fills the plate, while we leave the starches like rice, corn on the cob, and baked beans as side dishes. It is time to do an about face and think starches first, meat second, or sometimes not at all.

Starches get into fat trouble

Are starches healthy or not? The answer is yes, but. Grains, beans, and starchy vegetables start off healthy with plenty of energy, vitamins, and minerals. But then you load on the fats—butter on corn, cream cheese on a bagel, cream sauce on pasta, and potatoes deep-fried for french fries. Starches get in trouble because fat is added—in, on, and around.

The numbers show you how a healthy baked potato can go quickly from no fat to high fat:

1 medium baked potato = 160 calories, 0% calories from fat.
+2 tsp margarine = 90 calories, 100% calories from fat.
+2 Tbsp sour cream = 45 calories, 100% calories from fat.
Now the baked potato = 295 calories, 46% calories from fat.

In addition to the extra calories, some fats, such as butter, sour cream, and cream cheese, add the undesirables—saturated fat and cholesterol.

The starch challenges

You have two challenges. One, how to choose starches that contain little fat—roll or biscuit, fat-free crackers or butter crackers, steamed rice or fried rice. Two, how to seek out low- or no-fat toppers, such as tomato sauce, salsa, mustard, or low-fat sour cream. Let's go back to that baked potato for a moment. Hold the butter and drop a tablespoon or two of yogurt or fat-free sour cream flavored with garlic and herbs on top. That topper adds very few calories. You might want to try some others on the list of Low-Fat Starch Toppers on page 20.

Here are a few examples of high-fat and low-fat starches:

High-Fat Starches and Low-Fat Starches			
Food	Serving	Calories	Fat (g)
Muffin	1 3 oz	158	4
Bagel	1 3 oz	178	2
Croissant	1	109	6
Bread	1 slice	65	1
Potato chips	1 oz	152	10
Potato chips, fat free	1 oz	100	1
French fries	Small order	230	10
Baked potato	Small, 3 oz	98	0
Taco shell	1	100	6
Tortilla, corn	1	56	1
Macaroni and cheese	6 oz	250	13
Spaghetti and tomato sauce	6 oz	209	2
Refried beans	1/2 cup	136	3
Refried beans, fat free	1/2 cup	93	0

Starches and diabetes

The message: Eat more starches! That's the opposite of what you've heard for years. That's because research studies show it is healthiest for everyone to eat more grains, beans, and starchy vegetables. Starches are good for you because they have very little fat, saturated fat, or cholesterol. Yes, these foods do raise your blood glucose more quickly than meats and fats, so you may need to adjust your exercise or medication when you eat more of them.

Fiber and diabetes

Americans eat about half the amount of dietary fiber that we need. First, we do not eat enough grains, beans, starchy vegetables, or fruits and vegetables. Second, the fiber is processed out of food before we eat it. For example, whole wheat flour with the bran removed becomes white flour, and brown rice becomes white rice. Your first goal is to eat at least 20 g of fiber a day.

How many servings?

You should eat six or more servings a day. That might sound like a lot of starches, but you probably double up on servings without realizing it. For instance, you might make a sandwich with 2 slices of bread—that's 2 servings, or have 1 1/2 cups of pasta—that's 3 servings. The chart below suggests a number of servings of starches based on certain calorie levels.

	For weight loss for some women	Many older women	Many women, older adults	Older men, larger women	Kids, teen girls, active women, most men	Teen boys, active men
Calorie level	1200	1400	1600	1800	2200	2800
Servings	6	6	6	7	9	11

The sample 1-day meal plan on this page is used again in each of the following chapters. The nutrient information is only shown here. Check to see how easy it can be to eat 7 servings of starches in 1 day. The starches are in **bold** so that you can count them.

Breakfast
1 whole oat bran English muffin (2 servings)
1/2 large grapefruit
2 Tbsp light cream cheese

Lunch
1 pita pocket, 6" across, cut in half to fill (2 servings)
1/3 medium sliced tomato
1/3 cup sliced cucumbers
1/2 cup sliced large carrots or whole baby carrots
1 oz lean ham or turkey
1 oz part-skim Swiss cheese
Mustard to spread on bread
1 cup of low-fat/skim milk

Afternoon Snack
1 cup nonfat fruited yogurt sweetened with low-calorie sweetener
2 small tangerines

Dinner
5 oz dry red wine
1 cup spaghetti (2 servings)
1 whole wheat dinner roll (1 serving)
1 cup tomato sauce made with
    3/4 cup prepared tomato sauce
    1/3 cup onions
    1/3 cup peppers
    2 tsp canola oil (use to sauté onions and peppers)
    2 oz ground turkey, browned and drained (3 oz raw)
Spinach salad with
    1 cup spinach

1/3 cup sliced mushrooms

1 tsp purple onion

2 Tbsp reduced-fat French salad dressing

Evening Snack

1/2 cup light ice cream

1 1/4 cups whole strawberries, sliced

Sample 1-Day Meal Plan

Nutrition Facts

Calories 1850	
Total fat 48g,	**24% of calories**
Saturated 13g	
Monounsaturated 8g	
Cholesterol 99mg	
Sodium 3100mg	
Total carbohydrate 260g,	**57% of calories**
Dietary fiber 27g	
Sugars 75g	
Protein 80g,	**19% of calories**

Vitamin A	4163 RE	•	Vitamin C 371mg
Calcium	1333mg	•	Iron 13mg

A serving of starch

The chart on pages 22–28 shows serving sizes for some starches along with calories, fat, and fiber. Usually, one serving is 1/2 cup of cooked cereal, grain, pasta, or starchy vegetable, 1 oz of dry cereal, 1 oz (or slice in many cases) of bread, or 3/4–1 oz of most snack foods like pretzels or crackers. Each starch serving is roughly 15 g of carbohydrates, 3 g of protein, and 80 calories. These are the same numbers as starch exchanges. Remember, it is important to eat the correct serving size. Weigh and measure foods on occasion to make sure you're estimating correctly. Use the same bowls and cups to help you "eyeball" the amount. For example, eat cereal in the same bowl, serve pasta on the same plate.

Nutrition assets

In general, grains, beans, and starchy vegetables provide quick energy and are good sources of some B vitamins, magnesium, copper, iron, and dietary fiber. On the supermarket shelf, you'll find some starches that have had vitamins and minerals added at the factory. (See pages 159–162 for lists of foods to eat for many vitamins and minerals.)

Get to know yourself

If you want to change your eating habits, you need to know what you eat now. Ask yourself these questions:

▲ How many starch servings do I eat each day?

▲ What starches do I choose (is it a short or long list)?

▲ Do my starch choices have fat in, on, or around them?

▲ Do I eat high-fiber starches?

Change...one step at a time

Use your answers to the above questions to set your own goals. For instance, if you currently eat 6 servings of starch per day, but according to the chart on page 16 you should eat nine, then increase your starch servings gradually—the first month, try for 7, the next month 8, and so on. Try to eat starches without added fat. Remember that carbohydrate makes your blood glucose rise. Ask your health-care provider or dietitian for help adjusting your diabetes regimen to deal with this.

Easy ways to eat more grains, beans, and starchy vegetables

▲ In a meat loaf or meatball recipe, substitute some grain, such as bulgur or brown rice, for some of the meat.

▲ Add noodles, peas, or beans to a vegetable soup.

▲ Prepare a hearty bean or pea soup—divide the leftovers into individual portions, and store in the freezer for a quick meal.

▲ When you cook a grain, make enough for extra servings. You can toss it on salad, into soups or casseroles.

▲ Eat whole-grain cold cereal as a snack; pack the small boxes for snacks.

▲ Toss leftover cold corn, bulgur, or peas on a salad.

▲ Open a can of garbanzo beans (chickpeas) or kidney beans, and add them to a salad, tomato sauce, or three-bean salad.

▲ Treat yourself to great-tasting bread with meals, for a snack, or as the main course at breakfast.

▲ Add crunch to a salad or casserole with fat-free tortilla or potato chips.

▲ Have pretzels or light (in fat) popcorn for a snack.

Low-fat starch toppers

▲ Use reduced-calorie or fat-free cream cheese on bagels or toast.

▲ Put reduced-calorie or fat-free sour cream on potatoes.

▲ Blenderize cottage cheese and herbs or seasonings to put on pasta or baked potatoes.

▲ Put mustard on baked potatoes or sandwiches.

▲ Mix tomato sauce with pasta, rice, or grains.

▲ Use plain low-fat yogurt with or without herbs on baked potatoes. Mix plain yogurt with low-fat granola or other cold cereal.

▲ Use low-fat or fat-free mayonnaise for sandwiches.

▲ Put salsa on low-fat tortilla chips, Mexican burritos, or fajitas.

Now you know

▲ Eat more grains, beans, and starchy vegetables.

▲ Starchy foods are healthy for people with diabetes.

▲ Build meals from the base up. First decide on grains, beans, and starchy vegetables.

▲ Choose and prepare starches with little or no fat.

▲ Choose more starches with fiber in them.

Scenario

Meet Julie. She is 64 years old and has had type II diabetes for about 10 years. Julie has controlled her diabetes fairly well until recently. She has gained about 15 pounds over the last year, in part because she finally quit smoking. She was also very concerned about a granddaughter who was quite sick. Her doctor was pleased she quit smoking because her blood pressure was a bit lower. However, the doctor was concerned about her weight gain, especially because her glycated hemoglobin has been climbing. It is now 9.3%, which means her blood glucose levels average 200–300 mg/dl.

Julie recently started taking two types of insulin twice a day for better control. Her doctor suggested that she meet with an RD to help her get control of her weight and lower her blood glucose.

She worked with the RD to refocus her old meal plan. The dietitian suggested that Julie eat more starches and smaller amounts of protein and fat. So, instead of some meat at breakfast, Julie will try fruit, 2 starches, and a cup of skim milk and monitor her blood glucose. For her starches, Julie will trade off between a small bagel topped with light or fat-free cream cheese, dry cereal, oat bran, and on occasion, a frozen waffle with a small amount of maple syrup.

At lunch, she will decrease the amount of meat in her sandwich and get another starch and some crunch with fat-free tortilla chips, potato chips, or pretzels. Or she will toss garbanzo or kidney beans on a salad.

At dinner, she will try a few new recipes that have more starches—chili made with turkey sausage over a baked potato, a store-bought pizza with added vegetables, or pasta with a light, tomato-based meat sauce. This is certainly a switch for Julie, who remembers how she always tried to keep starches to a minimum.

	Serving	Calories	Carbo-hydrate (g)	Fat (g)	Fiber (g)
Cereal, cold					
All Bran	1/2 cup	75	22	1	10
Bran Buds	1/2 cup	112	33	1	16
Cheerios	3/4 cup	90	16	2	2
Cornflakes	3/4 cup	89	20	0	1
Fiber One	1/2 cup	60	24	1	13
40% Bran Flakes	1/2 cup	78	19	0	5
Granola, regular	1/4 cup	126	19	5	1
Granola, low-fat	1/4 cup	105	21	2	2
Grape-Nut Flakes	3/4 cup	104	24	0	3
Grape-Nuts	1/4 cup	105	24	0	3
Kix	3/4 cup	66	14	0	0
Muesli	1/4 cup	75	16	1	2
NutriGrain, wheat	1/2 cup	79	19	1	3
Product 19	3/4 cup	88	19	0	1
Puffed rice	1 1/2 cups	90	22	0	0
Puffed wheat	1 1/2 cups	76	15	0	1
Raisin Bran	1/2 cup	85	22	1	4
Rice Krispies	3/4 cup	71	16	0	0
Shredded Wheat	1/2 cup	90	20	1	3
Special K	3/4 cup	83	16	0	1
Sugar frosted cereal	1/2 cup	90	23	1	1
Sugar Frosted Flakes	1/2 cup	67	16	0	0
Total	3/4 cup	87	20	1	3
Wheat Chex	1/2 cup	85	19	1	2
Wheaties	3/4 cup	80	18	0	2
Cereals, hot, cooked					
Cream of rice	1/2 cup	63	14	0	0
Cream of wheat	1/2 cup	67	14	0	1
Cream of wheat, instant	1 pkt.	103	22	0	1

	Serving	Calories	Carbo-hydrate (g)	Fat (g)	Fiber (g)
Grits	1/2 cup	73	16	0	0
Maypo	1/2 cup	85	16	1	3
Oatmeal	1/2 cup	73	13	1	2
Oatmeal, instant	1 pkt.	94	18	2	3
Wheatena	1/2 cup	68	14	1	3
Whole wheat, cooked	1/2 cup	75	17	1	2

Grains

	Serving	Calories	Carbo-hydrate (g)	Fat (g)	Fiber (g)
Barley, cooked	1/3 cup	65	15	0	2
Bulgur, cooked	1/2 cup	76	17	0	4
Cornmeal, dry	3 Tbsp	97	21	1	2
Couscous, cooked	1/3 cup	67	14	0	1
Flour, white, all purpose	3 Tbsp	87	18	0	1
Flour, whole wheat	3 Tbsp	74	16	0	3
Macaroni, cooked	1/2 cup	99	20	1	1
Millet, cooked	1/4 cup	72	14	1	6
Noodles, egg, enriched, cooked	1/2 cup	106	20	1	1
Oatmeal, cooked	1/2 cup	72	13	1	5
Orzo	1/2 cup	98	20	1	1
Quinoa	1/2 cup	80	14	1	3
Rice, basmati, cooked	1/3 cup	75	16	2	—
Rice, brown, cooked	1/3 cup	72	15	1	1
Rice, white, long grain, cooked	1/3 cup	69	15	0	0
Rice milk	1/2 cup	85	19	2	—
Spaghetti, cooked	1/2 cup	99	20	1	1
Spinach pasta	1/2 cup	92	18	1	1
Wheat germ, toasted	3 Tbsp	80	10	2	3

	Serving	Calories	Carbo-hydrate (g)	Fat (g)	Fiber (g)
Bread					
Bagel	1/2	98	19	1	1
Biscuit, baked	1	127	17	6	1
Bran muffin, large, purchased	1/2	85	13	3	1
Bread, multigrain	1 slice	75	15	2	2
Bread, pumpernickel	1 slice	80	15	1	2
Bread, rye	1 slice	83	16	1	2
Bread, sourdough	1 slice	70	12	1	1
Bread, white, reduced calorie	2 slices	96	20	1	4
Bread, white (French, Italian)	1 slice	67	12	1	1
Bread, whole wheat	1 slice	70	13	1	2
Bread crumbs	1 Tbsp	60	11	1	0
Breadsticks	2 sticks	82	14	2	1
Cornbread, baked	2 oz	152	25	4	1
Croissant	1/2	115	13	6	1
English muffin	1/2	67	13	1	1
Hamburger bun	1/2	61	11	1	1
Hot dog bun	1/2	61	11	1	1
Muffin, baked, small, homemade	1	133	19	5	1
Muffin, purchased	1/2	133	19	5	1
Pancakes, from mix	2	166	22	6	1
Pita (6")	1/2	83	17	0	1
Raisin bread, unfrosted	1 slice	71	14	1	1
Roll, plain bread	1	85	14	2	1
Roll, whole wheat	1	90	15	2	1

	Serving	Calories	Carbo-hydrate (g)	Fat (g)	Fiber (g)
Stuffing, bread, purchased	1/3 cup	117	14	6	2
Taco shells	2	122	16	6	2
Tortilla, corn, 6–7" across	1	56	12	1	1
Tortilla, flour, 7–8" across	1	114	20	3	1
Waffle,	1	145	17	7	1
Waffle, 4 1/2" square, reduced fat	1	80	17	1	1

Crackers and Snacks

	Serving	Calories	Carbo-hydrate (g)	Fat (g)	Fiber (g)
Animal crackers	8	89	15	3	1
Butter-type crackers	6	90	11	5	0
Cheezits	24	140	14	8	—
Chow mein noodles	1/2 cup	116	13	2	1
Crispbread	2 slices	73	16	0	3
Crispbread, Wasa (Golden Rye)	2 slices	70	14	0	4
Croutons	1 cup	122	22	2	1
Graham crackers	3	89	16	2	1
Granola bar	1	133	18	6	2
Granola bar, fat free	1	140	35	0	3
Matzo	3/4 oz	83	18	0	1
Wheat cracker	7	112	14	5	1
Melba toast	4 slices	78	15	1	1
Oyster crackers	24	78	13	2	1
Popcorn, popped, no fat added	3 cups	92	19	1	4
Popcorn, microwave	3 cups	103	15	4	3
Popcorn, microwave, light	3 cups	65	11	2	2

	Serving	Calories	Carbo-hydrate (g)	Fat (g)	Fiber (g)
Potato chips	1 oz	152	15	10	1
Potato chips, fat free	23	82	17	0	2
Pretzels, hard, large	1 oz	110	23	1	—
Pretzels, sticks/rings	3/4 oz	80	17	1	1
Rice cake, regular	2	70	15	1	1
Rye crisp	3 slices	86	21	0	2
Saltine-type crackers	6	78	13	2	1
Saltine-type crackers, fat free	6	72	14	0	0
Sandwich crackers, cheese filling	3	99	13	5	0
Sandwich crackers, peanut butter filling	3	102	12	5	0
Tortilla chips, fried	1 oz	142	18	7	2
Tortilla chips, baked	17	82	18	1	3
Triscuits	6	128	18	6	2
Triscuits, reduced fat	5	81	15	2	3
Wheat Thins	12	105	14	5	2

Dried and Baked Beans, Peas, and Lentils

	Serving	Calories	Carbo-hydrate (g)	Fat (g)	Fiber (g)
Baked beans	1/3 cup	79	17	0	4
Baked beans, vegetarian	1/3 cup	79	16	1	4
Beans, fava, dried, cooked	1/2 cup	93	17	0	4
Beans, garbanzo, cooked	1/3 cup	95	15	2	3
Beans, kidney, canned, solids and liquid	1/3 cup	70	13	0	3
Beans, kidney, dried cooked	1/3 cup	74	13	0	4

	Serving	Calories	Carbo-hydrate (g)	Fat (g)	Fiber (g)
Beans, lima, canned, solids and liquids	1/2 cup	94	17	1	4
Beans, lima, frozen, cooked	1/2 cup	86	16	0	6
Beans, navy, dried, cooked	1/3 cup	85	16	1	5
Beans, pinto, dried, cooked	1/3 cup	78	15	0	5
Beans, white, dried, cooked	1/3 cup	83	15	0	4
Hummus	1/3 cup	140	17	7	3
Lentils, dried, cooked	1/2 cup	117	20	0	8
Peas, green, canned, drained	1/2 cup	59	11	0	4
Peas, green, frozen, cooked	1/2 cup	62	11	0	4
Peas, green, fresh, cooked	1/2 cup	67	13	0	2
Peas, split, dried, cooked	1/2 cup	117	21	0	8
Peas, black-eyed, dried, cooked	1/2 cup	100	18	0	6
Refried beans, fat free	1/2 cup	80	15	0	5

Starchy Vegetables

	Serving	Calories	Carbo-hydrate (g)	Fat (g)	Fiber (g)
Corn, frozen, cooked	1/2 cup	66	17	0	2
Corn, whole kernel, vacuum packed	1/2 cup	83	20	1	6
Corn on cob, cooked, medium	1	83	19	1	2

	Serving	Calories	Carbo-hydrate (g)	Fat (g)	Fiber (g)
Corn on cob, frozen, 3"	1	70	14	1	1
French fries, frozen, baked, no salt	20	120	20	4	2
Mixed vegetables with corn	1 cup	80	18	0	4
Mixed vegetables with pasta	1 cup	80	15	0	5
Parsnips, fresh, cooked	1/2 cup	63	15	2	4
Plantain, cooked, slices	1/2 cup	89	24	0	2
Potato, baked, with skin	3 oz	93	22	0	2
Potato, white, boiled, peeled	3 oz	73	17	0	2
Potato, mashed, flakes (with milk and fat)	1/2 cup	119	16	6	2
Potato, sweet, canned, vacuum packed, pieces	1/2 cup	92	22	0	3
Squash, winter, acorn, or butternut	1 cup	83	22	0	7
Yam, plain	1/2 cup	79	19	0	2

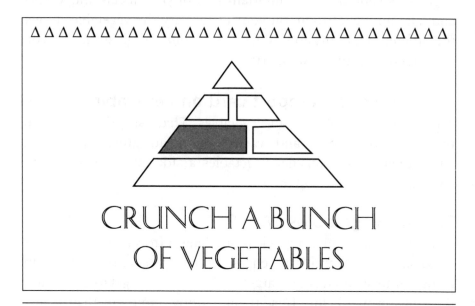

△ △

CHAPTER 4

CRUNCH A BUNCH OF VEGETABLES

What you will learn

▲ How many servings of vegetables you should eat each day.
▲ Proper serving sizes of vegetables.
▲ Easy ways to crunch more vegetables.

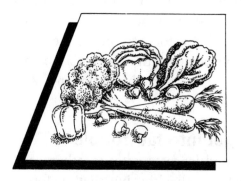

Next up: vegetables

Look at the food pyramid. Vegetables are in the section right above grains, beans, and starchy vegetables and next to fruits. This is the second largest space on the pyramid. The pyramid tells you to eat 3–5 servings per day (the largest number of servings after starches).

Vegetables should be an important part of your meals and snacks and take up lots of room on your plate. Vary the vegetables to get the different vitamins and minerals they offer. Vegetables give you a lot of crunch for a few calories.

America's report card on vegetables

Americans don't eat enough vegetables. That's surprising with all the fresh vegetables and variety of salad greens available. Unfortunately, we consider vegetables a side dish, not the main course.

Too few vegetables: Why?

When we prepare meals quickly—perhaps a frozen chicken entree or package of macaroni and cheese—we don't take time to cut up a salad or to steam fresh asparagus. "I don't buy vegetables because they turn brown before I use them. I throw more out than I eat." This is a chicken and egg argument. If you do not buy vegetables, you cannot eat them. But, if you eat them, they cannot go bad.

Restaurant eating and eating on the run don't include many vegetables. It is just not as easy to wolf down a salad in your car as it is a burger and fries. More pizzas are topped with pepperoni and extra cheese than onions, mushrooms, and peppers. In fancy restaurants, your plate may be delivered with tiny vegetable portions because the chef is focused on the meat. You might not even ask what vegetable comes with a particular main course. It's easy to understand why we have trouble following Mom's advice to "eat your vegetables."

Vegetables get into fat trouble

Just as starches and fat taste good together, so do vegetables and fat. Yes, vegetables are healthy, but that's before you douse lettuce greens with blue cheese dressing, cover green beans with cream of mushroom soup and fried onion rings, or order fried zucchini appetizers. Fat adds unhealthy calories.

Here are the numbers to show how a healthy helping of broccoli quickly becomes unhealthy with added fat in the cheese sauce.

1 cup cooked broccoli = 44 calories, 0% calories from fat

2 Tbsp cheese sauce (4 g fat) = 36 calories

1 cup broccoli and cheese sauce = 80 calories, 45% calories from fat

Here are a few more examples of what fat adds to vegetables:

Higher-fat and lower-fat vegetables Food	Serving	Calories	Fat (g)
Fried zucchini, breaded and deep-fried	1/2 cup	279	16
Sauteed zucchini with broth and sherry	1/2 cup	30	0
Green bean casserole	1/2 cup	160	11
Green beans steamed with garlic and herbs	1/2 cup	22	0
Spinach souffle	1/2 cup	110	9
Spinach and vinegar	1/2 cup	20	0
Salad	1 cup salad		
with regular blue cheese dressing	2 Tbsp	191	16
Salad	1 cup salad		
with fat-free blue cheese dressing	2 Tbsp	57	0

Do you hide vegetables under cream sauce? Do you dunk raw vegetables in a sour cream or mayonnaise dip? Your challenge is to find ways to prepare and eat vegetables with little fat. Make changes one at a time. For example, put butter or margarine on the table and let family members choose how much they want. Slice a fresh lemon or lime into wedges to squeeze on steamed broccoli, or sprinkle cinnamon or nutmeg in the water when you microwave sliced carrots. These ideas add flavor with no fat.

Salad and Dressing—Famous Pals

Perhaps the most famous vegetable and fat combo is salad and dressing. You select a low-calorie and no-fat salad with greens, tomatoes, cucumbers, etc. Then you pour on a couple of table-spoons of regular salad dressing. This can add 150 calories of pure fat. The challenge is to keep salads nutrient rich and fat poor. Watch other high-fat toppings, such as cheese, pasta or potato salad, olives, or sunflower seeds.

Salad Dressing Know-How

Your choice of salad dressings is wider than ever. The only down-side is the time it takes to read all the labels. You have regular, reduced fat, low calorie, fat free, and homemade. Just remember that the terms *reduced fat* and *fat free* do not mean *calorie free*. Here is the nutrition lowdown on three varieties of two favorite dressings:

	Calories*	Carbohydrate (g)	Fat (g)
Thousand Island			
Regular	118	5	11
Low calorie	48	5	3
Fat free	20	6	0
Italian			
Regular	183	2	20
Low calorie	32	2	3
Fat free	18	4	0

*All 2 Tbsp servings

Note that your choices can make the calories go down, but all salad dressings have calories.

Here are a few other tricks with salad dressing. These come in handy, especially when you eat away from home.

▲ Ask for reduced-calorie or fat-free dressings.

▲ Order salad dressing on the side.

▲ Request a light or small amount of dressing on the salad.

▲ Request some vinegar or lemon wedges on the side to dilute the small amount of dressing.

▲ Do not overload the salad with dressing. (Hint: if you always find dressing at the bottom of your salad, you can use less.)

Vegetables and diabetes

For people with diabetes, it's "the more the merrier" when it comes to vegetables. Eat at least 3 servings a day. Vegetables are healthy, chock full of vitamins and minerals, and some have fiber. The best part: vegetables are naturally low in calories.

How many servings

Three to five servings a day. Vegetables are the one food that you can eat a lot of because they add so few calories and don't raise blood glucose very much. The chart below gives some suggestions for the number of servings to eat based on your calorie range.

	For weight loss for some women	Many older women	Many women, older adults	Older men, larger women	Kids, teen girls, active women, most men	Teen boys, active men
Calorie level	1200	1400	1600	1800	2200	2800
Servings	3	3	3	4	4	5

Check the sample menu to see how vegetables can add up. The nutrient information is on page 18. The vegetables are in **bold** type.

Breakfast
1 whole oat bran English muffin
1/2 large grapefruit
2 Tbsp light cream cheese

Lunch

1 pita pocket, 6" across, cut in half to fill
1/3 medium sliced tomato (1/2 serving)
1/3 cup sliced cucumbers (1/2 serving)
1/2 cup sliced large carrots or whole baby carrots (1/2 serving)
1 oz lean ham or turkey
1 oz part-skim Swiss cheese
Mustard to spread on bread
1 cup of low-fat/skim milk

Afternoon Snack

1 cup nonfat fruited yogurt sweetened with low-calorie sweetener
2 small tangerines

Dinner

5 oz dry red wine
1 cup spaghetti
1 whole wheat dinner roll
1 cup tomato sauce made with
    3/4 cup prepared tomato sauce (1 1/2 servings)
    1/3 cup onions (1/3 serving)
    1/3 cup peppers (1/3 serving)
    2 tsp canola oil (use to sauté onions and peppers)
    2 oz ground turkey, browned and drained (3 oz raw)
Spinach salad with
    1 cup spinach (1 serving)
    1/3 cup sliced mushrooms (1/3 serving)
    1 tsp purple onion
    2 Tbsp reduced-fat French salad dressing

Evening Snack

1/2 cup light ice cream
1 1/4 cups whole strawberries, sliced

A serving of vegetables

The chart at the end of the chapter shows serving sizes for many common vegetables plus their nutrition profile. In general, 1 serving is 1 cup of raw vegetables or 1/2 cup of cooked vegetables. Each vegetable serving is about 5 g of carbohydrates, 2 g of protein, and 25 calories. These numbers are the same as vegetable exchanges. Remember, it is important to eat the correct amount, so weigh and measure your foods.

Nutrition assets

The few calories in vegetables come from carbohydrate and a small amount of protein. Vegetables are good sources of fiber, vitamins such as A, beta-carotene (a form of vitamin A), C, and K and minerals such as calcium and magnesium. Different vegetables offer different vitamins and minerals. For instance, the dark green leafy vegetables, such as kale, are good sources of calcium, but yellow vegetables, such as carrots, are good sources of vitamin A.

Eat more raw

An easy way to eat more vegetables is to eat them raw—a few stalks of broccoli or cauliflower, a handful of cherry tomatoes, or sticks of zucchini. If you eat raw vegetables, you don't lose vitamins and minerals to cooking. Stock the refrigerator with a ready-to-go supply of vegetables, and have a handful for lunch, dinner, or snack. If you do not like some vegetables raw but you will eat them cooked and chilled, blanch a bunch of green beans, head of broccoli, or handful of snow peas. Stash them in a plastic container in the refrigerator ready to eat.

To blanch vegetables, boil a small amount of water with a pinch of salt, and steam vegetables for 2–3 minutes. Vegetables should be slightly soft but still crisp. Remove the pot from the stove or microwave, and place the vegetables in ice water.

Starches and vegetables go together

The food pyramid says to build meals around starches and vegetables. Try stir-fried vegetables and brown rice, tomato sauce with sautéed vegetables and pasta, vegetarian pizza, vegetarian lasagna, and cold marinated rice and diced vegetable salad served over greens.

Get to know yourself

If you want to change your eating habits, learn what you eat now. Ask these questions:

▲ How many vegetable servings do I eat a day?

▲ What vegetables do I eat (a narrow list or a wide variety)?

▲ Do I eat some raw vegetables every day?

▲ Do I add or prepare vegetables with fat?

Change...one step at a time

Using your answers to the questions above, set one goal at a time. How many vegetables should you eat each day? If you do well to eat two vegetable servings a day and you should have four, think up ways to eat more. Can you eat a double portion at dinner, have a handful of blanched broccoli as a snack or to pack with lunch? Put vegetables on center stage for lunch or dinner—a big salad at lunch or a stir-fry of vegetables at dinner. Find new ways to eat and prepare vegetables that are tasty but lower in fat.

Easy ways to eat your vegetables

▲ Keep some frozen and canned vegetables on hand so you always have vegetables ready.

▲ Make double and triple portions—eat a serving one day and have another one ready to go for the next.

▲ Blanch (quick cook and chill) a head of broccoli or cauliflower, break it into pieces, place it in a plastic container, and have a ready supply for the week, hot or cold.

▲ Keep a bag of baby carrots around—have a handful as a snack, pack them with lunch, add them to stew, microwave for a quick dish.

▲ Microwave or sauté onions and peppers to put more vegetables into a tomato sauce.

▲ Put extra vegetables on a frozen pizza.

▲ Make a big salad to last a few days, store in a plastic container.

▲ Remember, almost anything healthy can top a salad—green peas, bulgur, leftover rice, garbanzo beans, green beans, Grape-Nuts, raisins, pineapple, dried apricots. Let your imagination flow.

▲ Add vegetables to sandwiches—not just the old lettuce and tomato. Try alfalfa sprouts, sliced red onion, sliced cucumbers, sliced yellow squash or zucchini, red peppers.

▲ Add vegetables to an omelette or scrambled eggs—sauté onions, peppers, mushrooms, tomatoes, and add some fresh herbs.

▲ Drink tomato or V8 juice, or Bloody Mary mix. (Watch the sodium.)

▲ In a tomato sauce, cut the amount of meat you use in half and add more vegetables—onions, peppers, mushrooms, eggplant, zucchini, or others.

Now you know

▲ You should eat 3–5 servings of vegetables each day.

▲ Vegetables are important low-calorie sources of vitamins and minerals.

▲ Limit fats when preparing and eating vegetables.

▲ Quick and easy ways to eat more vegetables.

Scenario

Meet Brent. He is 25 years old, has had type I diabetes for 7 years, and takes insulin three times a day. He tries to regulate his blood glucose tightly because he wants to prevent diabetes complications, especially losing his eyesight. He is physically active with his company's softball team and works out in a gym three times a week.

Brent eats 2500–3000 calories a day to keep his weight between 177 and 180 pounds. He recently read that people should eat 5 servings of fruit and vegetables a day. He only gets 2–3 vegetable servings a day—lettuce and tomato on a hamburger at lunch, a salad, or maybe frozen spinach souffle or broccoli with cheese sauce at dinner. During a recent visit with a dietitian, he set 4–5 servings of vegetables and fruits as his daily goal.

Brent and his RD strategized ways to fit more vegetables in each day. When he takes lunch to work, he will put some slices of cucumber and alfalfa sprouts on his sandwiches and take baby carrots or red pepper slices to eat along with his sandwich. When he eats in a restaurant or cafeteria, he'll request extra lettuce, tomato, and onion on a sandwich and make a salad from the salad bar, or have a hot vegetable. He will try to keep frozen vegetables in the freezer and include a double helping of one at dinner.

He will try to buy lower-fat frozen vegetables without butter, cream, and cheese sauces. To add flavor to steamed vegetables, he will use fresh lemon or lime and only a small amount of butter.

When he has pizza for dinner—a couple times a week—he will hold the extra cheese and ground meat and request sliced tomato, onions, and mushrooms instead. He likes vegetable toppings, they're just not the usual when he orders pizza with friends. He will keep individual cans of V8 and Bloody Mary mix at home and in his desk at work to drink as a vegetable when he is in a pinch.

At the end of each Monday and Tuesday for the next 4 weeks, he will make a note of how many vegetable servings he ate that day and mark that in his calendar. This will help him chart his progress.

	Serving	Calories	Carbo-hydrate (g)	Fiber (g)
Vegetables, cooked, fresh, frozen, or canned				
Artichoke	1/2	30	7	3
Artichoke hearts, in water	1/2 cup	36	7	1
Asparagus, fresh or frozen	1/2 cup	23	4	3
Asparagus, spears, canned	1/2 cup	23	3	2
Bamboo shoots, canned	1/2 cup	15	3	1
Beans (green, wax, Italian)				
canned, drained	1/2 cup	14	3	1
Beets, canned	1/2 cup	26	6	2
Bok choy, Chinese				
cabbage	1/2 cup	10	2	1
Broccoli	1/2 cup	26	5	3
Brussels sprouts	1/2 cup	33	7	3
Cabbage	1/2 cup	16	3	2
Carrots	1/2 cup	35	8	3
Carrots, canned, drained	1/2 cup	17	4	1
Cauliflower	1/2 cup	17	3	2
Celery	1/2 cup	14	3	1
Eggplant	1/2 cup	13	3	1
Greens				
Beet greens	1/2 cup	20	4	2
Collard greens	1/2 cup	17	4	1
Kale	1/2 cup	21	4	1
Mustard greens	1/2 cup	10	2	1
Turnip greens	1/2 cup	14	3	2
Leeks	1/2 cup	16	4	2
Mushrooms	1/2 cup	21	4	2
Okra	1/2 cup	34	8	3
Onions, chopped	1/2 cup	46	11	2
Pasta sauce, canned				
(check sodium)	1/2 cup	110	17	4
Pea pods	1/2 cup	34	6	2
Peppers, green, red,				
or yellow	1/2 cup	19	5	1

	Serving	Calories	Carbo-hydrate (g)	Fiber (g)
Sauerkraut (sodium)	1/2 cup	22	5	3
Spaghetti sauce (sodium)	1/2 cup	136	20	4
Spinach	1/2 cup	27	5	3
Squash, summer	1/2 cup	18	4	1
Swiss chard	1/2 cup	18	4	2
Tomato sauce (sodium)	1/2 cup	37	9	2
Tomatoes, canned	1/2 cup	24	5	1
Tomato juice (sodium)	1/2 cup	21	5	1
Turnips, cubed	1/2 cup	14	4	2
Vegetable juice (sodium)	1/2 cup	23	6	1
Water chestnuts	1/2 cup	35	9	2
Zucchini	1/2 cup	14	4	1

Vegetables, raw

	Serving	Calories	Carbo-hydrate (g)	Fiber (g)
Alfalfa sprouts	1 cup	8	2	1
Bean sprouts	1 cup	31	6	2
Cabbage, Chinese	1 cup	12	3	1
Cabbage, green	1 cup	18	4	2
Carrots	1 cup	47	11	3
Cauliflower	1 cup	25	5	3
Celery	1 cup	19	4	2
Cucumber	1 cup	14	3	1
Mushrooms	1 cup	18	3	1
Onion	1 cup	61	14	3
Onion, green	1 cup	32	7	3
Pea pods	1 cup	61	11	4
Pepper, green	1 cup	27	6	2
Pepper, hot green chili	1 cup	60	14	2
Radishes	1 cup	20	4	2
Salad greens	1 cup	9	1	1
Spinach	1 cup	12	2	2
Squash, summer	1 cup	26	6	3
Tomato, chopped	1 cup	38	8	2
Tomato, small	1	26	6	2
Zucchini	1 cup	18	4	2

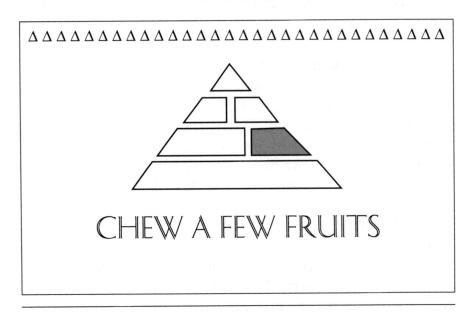

CHAPTER 5

CHEW A FEW FRUITS

What you will learn

▲ The number of servings of fruits you should eat each day.

▲ Proper serving sizes of fruit.

▲ Easy ways to eat more fruit.

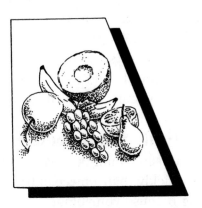

Side by side

On the food pyramid, fruits sit next to vegetables in the third-largest space. The pyramid tells you to eat 3–4 servings per day. Fruits are important for several reasons. They are good sources of vitamins, minerals, and fiber. Fruit contains no fat and may satisfy a sweet tooth. You have great choices from apples to watermelons.

America's report card on fruits

We get a failing grade on fruits (just as we do for vegetables and starches) because we do not eat enough of them. The foods that should be the foundation of your pyramid—starches, vegetables, and fruit—have been passed over for meats, fats, and sweets. That way of eating has the pyramid turned upside down. Fruit is often an afterthought, if we remember to eat it at all.

Too little fruit

Our excuses for not eating enough fruit are similar to the excuses for not eating our vegetables. "Too much trouble, don't have any around when I'm hungry." Interestingly, in our fast-paced world, fruit is an ideal food—no preparation, just wash, peel, and eat.

Too often, however, fruit is left to rot. We find it easier to buy candy bars, potato chips, or sandwich crackers. Why? Do you find pieces of fruit for sale in a convenience store, coffee shop, or bagel stop, fast food, or upscale restaurant? Not often.

You might not bring fresh fruit home because it gets soft and brown before you eat it. Then you don't have fruit in the house when you want it. Or you don't eat breakfast at home, so you miss the ripe opportunity for a few slices of banana or peaches on cereal or raisins in your oatmeal. And when it comes to a late-night sweet, ice cream, frozen yogurt, or custard wins out.

Fruit and diabetes

Questions about fruit keep coming up. Will fruit juice raise blood glucose levels more quickly than a piece of fruit? Should you avoid fruit in the morning because your blood glucose might be higher than at other times in the day? Is it better to eat fruit with meals rather than snacks?

All carbohydrates, whether rice, potatoes, or fruit juice, raise blood glucose about the same. In general, an equal amount of carbohydrate (15 g), such as 1/2 cup of grapefruit juice or 4 slices of

Melba toast, should raise blood glucose at about the same speed and to about the same degree.

However, that varies based on several factors: whether you eat a piece of fruit after a high-fat meal or sip fruit juice on an empty stomach, what your blood glucose is when you eat the fruit, whether the fruit is cooked or raw, how much diabetes medication you have in your body, etc. Also, people have individual differences.

So, your challenge is to determine how fruit works in your body. Does eating fruit in the morning make it more difficult for you to keep your blood glucose controlled throughout the day? Does one particular kind of fruit send your blood glucose soaring? Or does a piece of fruit as an afternoon snack give you just enough carbohydrate to last until dinner?

Eat fruit each day for vitamins and minerals. Be honest with yourself about your serving sizes. It is easy to drink a few extra ounces of fruit juice or to call a huge piece of fruit 1 serving when it is really 2. Use blood glucose monitoring to answer your questions about how fruit works in your body. The steps to take to track your response to fruit are: check the serving size, eat your fruit, and check your blood glucose level.

How many servings

You should eat three to four servings a day. That number can be hard to reach. But you can focus on eating a *combination* of at least 5 servings of fruits and vegetables each day. (If you eat 3 vegetables and 2 fruits, you're doing great.)

On the other hand, you might be overeating fruit. The calories add up quickly, especially if your portions are large. Consider a large apple (8 oz) at 140 calories versus a small apple (4 oz) at about 60 calories. That is 80 calories more for *one* apple. If you do that several times a day or week, you may gain weight or upset your blood glucose control.

The chart on the next page gives the specific number of servings to eat based on your calorie range.

	For weight loss for some women	Many older women	Many women, older adults	Older men, larger women	Kids, teen girls, active women, most men	Teen boys, active men
Calorie level	1200	1400	1600	1800	2200	2800
Servings	3	3	3	3	4	4

Look at this sample meal plan to see how easy it is to fit in 3 servings of fruits. The nutrient information is on page 18. Fruits are in **bold** so you can count them.

Breakfast
    1 whole oat bran English muffin
    1/2 large grapefruit (1 serving)
    2 Tbsp light cream cheese

Lunch
    1 pita pocket, 6" across, cut in half to fill
    1/3 medium sliced tomato
    1/3 cup sliced cucumbers
    1/2 cup sliced large carrots or whole baby carrots
    1 oz lean ham or turkey
    1 oz part-skim Swiss cheese
    Mustard to spread on bread
    1 cup of low-fat/skim milk

Afternoon Snack
    1 cup nonfat fruited yogurt sweetened with low-calorie sweetener
    2 small tangerines (1 serving)

Dinner
    5 oz dry red wine

1 cup spaghetti
1 whole wheat dinner roll
1 cup tomato sauce made with
    3/4 cup prepared tomato sauce
    1/3 cup onions
    1/3 cup peppers
    2 tsp canola oil (use to sauté onions and peppers)
    2 oz ground turkey, browned and drained (3 oz raw)
Spinach salad with
    1 cup spinach
    1/3 cup sliced mushrooms
    1 tsp purple onion
    2 Tbsp reduced-fat French salad dressing

Evening Snack
    1/2 cup light ice cream
    1 1/4 cups whole strawberries, sliced (1 serving)

A serving of fruit

The chart at the end of this chapter shows the serving size for many common fruits along with their nutrition profile. In general, you can think of 1 serving as 1 small to medium-sized fresh fruit; 1/2 cup of canned or fresh fruit, or fruit juice; or 1/4 cup of dried fruit. Pay careful attention to the portions. Each fruit serving has about 15 g of carbohydrates and 60 calories. This is the same as a fruit exchange.

Remember, the calories from fruit quickly add up. Weigh and measure fruit to make sure you estimate correctly. See what a 4-, 6-, and 8-oz apple looks like. Keep that in mind when you shop.

Nutrition assets

The calories from fruit are almost totally carbohydrate. Fruits have zero fat, except in some desserts. Fruits are excellent sources of some vitamins, such as A and C, and minerals, such as potassium, magnesium, and copper. For more about vitamins and minerals, see pages 158–162.

Dress fruit up for dessert

Fruit makes a great dessert, from apple cobbler to key lime pie. The problem is that many grams of fat, carbohydrate, and calories come along too. Here are a few examples of what happens to fruits when they become dessert:

High- and low-calorie dessert choices

Food	Serving	Calories	Fat (g)
Apple crisp	1 cup	194	8
Apple, peeled and baked with low-calorie sweetener and cinnamon	1	73	0
Banana cream pie	1 piece	398	20
Banana bread	1 slice	120	5
Strawberry ice cream	1 cup	254	11
Strawberries (frozen) on angel food cake	1/2 cup 1 piece	194	0

Your challenge is to search for ways to prepare fruits to satisfy your sweet tooth but not add a notch to your belt buckle. Here are a few quick ideas to start you off:

▲ Baked apples, low-calorie apple cobbler, or applesauce

▲ Banana bread, frozen bananas rolled in cocoa

▲ Sliced bananas or canned peaches or pears in fat-free, sugar-free pudding mix

▲ Frozen (no-sugar-added) blueberries or strawberries on frozen yogurt or topped with plain yogurt

▲ Frozen (no-sugar-added) blueberries or strawberries on angel food cake

▲ Sliced fresh fruit or fruit kabobs dipped in fruited yogurt or other low-calorie dip

▲ Strawberries, raspberries, or blueberries marinated in balsamic vinegar and served over frozen yogurt or angel food cake

▲ Peaches, nectarines, or oranges marinated in sherry or liqueur

and served over light ice cream
▲ Marinate fresh fruit in sherry or liqueur and place on skewers, serve with main course or as dessert (you can grill fruit on skewers also)

Juice, punch, or seltzer

Fruit punch, fruited iced tea, carbonated fruit drinks, and flavored seltzer masquerade as healthy. Reality is that these drinks are nothing more than sugar water or high-fructose corn syrup and water. They are not one bit healthier than regular soda even when they contain a splash of fruit juice. Here are the facts on new-age beverages:

New-Age Beverages		
Beverage (8 oz)*	**Calories**	**Carbohydrate (g)**
Kiwi strawberry fruit drink	130	33
Fruit punch drink	117	30
Iced tea, fruit flavored	110	27
Regular soda, cola type, (for comparison)	101	26

*This is the reference portion; however, most beverages are bottled in at least 12-oz servings.

According to food-labeling laws, a manufacturer can only use the term *fruit juice* if the product is 100% fruit juice. A *fruit drink* has only 10% fruit juice. Manufacturers must put the percentage of fruit juice in the product on the label. Purchase only 100% juice. You should get all the vitamins and minerals you can from those calories rather than just empty sugar calories.

Try these no-calorie thirst quenchers: water, mineral water, flavored mineral water (no calories), iced tea (unsweetened or sweetened with low-calorie sweetener), powdered beverage mix with low-calorie sweetener (e.g., Crystal Light), club soda, diet soda, hot tea, or hot coffee.

Get to know yourself

If you want to change your eating habits, you need to know what and how you eat now. Ask yourself these questions:

▲ How many fruit servings do I eat a day?

▲ Do I weigh portions of fruit? Are they the correct portion or larger?

▲ What fruits do I choose (a narrow group or wide variety)?

▲ What do I drink to quench my thirst?

▲ Do I drink fruit juice? Do I measure the amount?

▲ Does fruit cause me problems with blood glucose control?

Change...one step at a time

Your answers to the above questions can help you set your goals toward healthy eating. Do you need to eat more fruit servings? What keeps you from eating fruit? Is it in the house, in restaurants you go to? You can take a piece of fruit to eat in the afternoon or toss a couple of tablespoons of raisins on your breakfast cereal. It's better to get your fruit calories from pieces of fruit rather than fruit juice. Fruit has fiber and is more filling. Remember, 5 a day for fruits and vegetables.

Easy ways to eat more fruit

▲ Add slices of banana or peaches to cold cereal.

▲ Add raisins, pieces of dried apricot, or apple when cooking hot cereal.

▲ Keep a plastic container full of cut-up fruit so you can have some at breakfast or for a snack topped with plain or fruited low-fat yogurt (for more calcium).

▲ Take 1 or 2 pieces of fruit from home each day to eat with lunch, as an afternoon snack, or on your way home to take the edge off your hunger.

▲ Keep dried fruit, raisins, figs, apricots, peaches, pears, etc., around to use for a snack, for fuel on long hikes or bike rides, or to stash in your desk or locker (watch your serving size).

▲ Put a few raisins, pieces of apple or dried apricot, or pineapple chunks on a salad.

▲ Keep canned or jarred fruit in the pantry—applesauce, peaches, pears, and pineapple for starters.

▲ Toss fruit into entrees—pineapple in stir-fry or on pizza, fresh or dried cranberries or peaches in chicken dishes, or apricots or apples in pork dishes.

▲ Combine fruit with vegetables—crushed pineapple in coleslaw; raisins in carrot salad; Waldorf salad with apples, raisins, walnuts, and celery.

▲ Serve fruit with the main course—applesauce with pork chops or roast, pineapple with ham, homemade cranberry sauce with chicken.

▲ Grill fruit on skewers and serve as dessert with a few ginger snaps or vanilla wafers, or serve as part of the main course.

Now you know

▲ How much fruit to eat each day.

▲ Importance of being precise about your portions of fruit.

▲ The vitamins and minerals fruit offers.

▲ Quick and easy ways to eat more fruits.

Scenario

Meet David. He is 38 years old and has had type II diabetes for 8 years. When he was diagnosed, he was told to eat healthy foods and to avoid too many sweets. Recently, he began to have some vision problems and was feeling symptoms of thirst and tiredness.

His doctor found that his blood glucose was high, and his glycated hemoglobin was 9.4. This means that his blood glucose has been averaging around 220 mg/dl. His blood pressure was also high, 195/90 mm/hg. David's physician suggested that he begin taking a diabetes medication to lower his blood glucose and a blood pressure medication. He gave him a list of dietitians who could help him trim off a few pounds and cut back on sodium.

David and the dietitian discussed what he usually eats and drinks, and David was surprised to see what his food "habits" are. David is a construction worker and, in the warm climate, gets thirsty on the job. He has been drinking fruit-flavored seltzers and sports drinks to quench his thirst. He has been eating 1 fruit a day—maybe a small banana on a bowl of cereal. But David said he eats a plain donut or two and a cup of coffee in his truck on the way to the job. He might then eat a piece of fruit in the evening.

David's dietitian explained that these fruit and sports drinks have a lot of sugar and not much in the way of nutrition. She suggested that he quench his thirst with water, mineral water, iced tea, or diet lemonade.

The RD gave David the idea of cutting up grapefruits, apples, oranges, and pears and putting them in a plastic container in the refrigerator. Then he would have ready access to fruit salad. She suggested he put a few tablespoons of nonfat, sugar-free fruited yogurt on for extra taste and calcium. To increase the number of fruits per day, David said he'd be willing to eat a piece of fruit before he leaves for work and keep servings of dried fruit in his glove compartment to eat one serving in the afternoon. He will try for a third fruit as part of an evening snack of cereal and milk or yogurt and ginger snaps.

	Serving	Calories	Carbo-hydrate (g)	Fiber (g)
Fruit, fresh				
Apple, unpeeled, small	1	63	16	3
Apricots	4	68	16	3
Banana, small	1	64	16	2
Blackberries	3/4 cup	56	14	5
Blueberries	3/4 cup	61	15	3
Cantaloupe	1 cup	56	13	1
Cherries, sweet	12	59	14	2
Cranberries	1 cup	47	12	4
Figs, large	1 1/2	71	18	3
Grapefruit	1/2	51	13	2
Grapes, seedless	17	60	15	1
Honeydew melon	1 cup	59	16	1
Kiwi	1	56	14	3
Mango	1/2 cup	68	18	2
Nectarine	1	67	16	2
Orange	1	62	15	3
Papaya	1 cup	55	14	3
Peach, medium	1	57	15	3
Pear, large	1/2	59	15	2
Pineapple	3/4 cup	57	14	1
Plums, small	2	73	17	2
Raspberries, black, red	1 cup	60	14	8
Rhubarb	2 cups	52	11	4
Strawberries	1 1/4 cups	56	13	4
Tangerine, small	2	74	19	3
Watermelon, cubed	1 1/4 cups	64	14	1
Fruit, canned, jarred, juice packed				
Applesauce, unsweetened	1/2 cup	52	14	2
Apricots	1/2 cup	60	15	2
Cherries, sweet, juice packed	1/2 cup	68	17	1
Cranberry sauce	1/4 cup	86	22	1
Fruit cocktail, juice packed	1/2 cup	57	15	1
Fruit cocktail	1/2 cup	55	14	1

	Serving	Calories	Carbo-hydrate (g)	Fiber (g)
Grapefruit, juice packed	3/4 cup	69	17	1
Mandarin oranges	3/4 cup	69	18	1
Peaches, juice packed	1/2 cup	55	14	1
Pears, juice packed	1/2 cup	62	16	3
Pineapple, juice packed	1/2 cup	74	20	1
Plums, juice packed	1/2 cup	73	19	1
Pumpkin, solid packed	3/4 cup	59	15	6
Fruit, dried				
Apples, rings	4	63	17	2
Apricots, halves	8	66	17	3
Dates	3	68	18	2
Figs	1 1/2	71	18	3
Fruit snacks, chewy, roll	1	78	18	1
Prunes, uncooked	3	60	16	2
Raisins, dark, seedless	2 Tbsp	54	14	1

Fruit, frozen unsweetened

	Serving	Calories	Carbo-hydrate (g)	Fiber (g)
Blackberries	3/4 cup	73	18	6
Blueberries	3/4 cup	58	14	3
Melon balls	1 cup	57	14	1
Raspberries	1/2 cup	61	15	6
Strawberries	1 1/4 cups	65	17	4
Fruit juices				
Apple juice/cider	1/2 cup	58	15	0
Apricot nectar	1/2 cup	70	17	0
Cranapple juice cocktail	1/3 cup	53	13	0
Cranberry juice cocktail	1/3 cup	48	12	0
Fruit juice bars, 100% juice	1	75	19	0
Grape juice	1/3 cup	51	13	0
Orange juice, canned	1/2 cup	52	12	0
Orange juice, fresh	1/2 cup	56	13	0
Orange juice, frozen	1/2 cup	56	13	0
Pineapple juice, canned	1/2 cup	70	17	0
Prune juice	1/3 cup	60	15	1

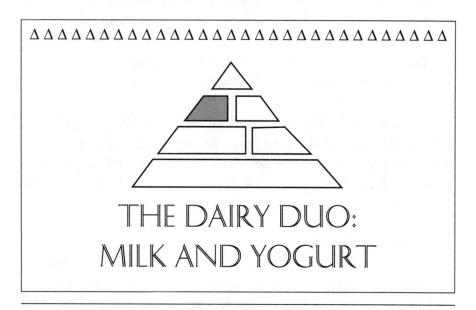

CHAPTER 6

THE DAIRY DUO: MILK AND YOGURT

What you will learn

▲ The number of servings of milk and yogurt to eat each day.
▲ Proper serving sizes of milk and yogurt.
▲ Easy ways to get more milk and yogurt.

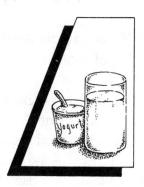

As the pyramid narrows

As the pyramid slims toward the top, we find milk. Milk takes up the same amount of space as meat and others (protein foods). They have much less room than grains, beans, and starchy vegetables; vegetables; and fruits. In the Diabetes Food Pyramid, the milk group contains all types of milk and yogurt, but cheese is in the meat group. So, what does this pyramid tell you about milk? Have 2–3 servings per day. Milk and yogurt provide nutrients you need, especially calcium, and if you select skim, fat-free, and low-fat milk and yogurt, you can hold the fat count close to zero.

America's report card on milk and yogurt

Milk's little space on the food pyramid might tell you to limit milk and yogurt. But, if you are like most Americans, you should have more—fat-free and low-fat types. Most Americans do not consume enough dairy foods to meet their calcium needs.

Not enough milk

You think of milk and yogurt as foods you buy at the supermarket and eat only at home. You stop at a convenience store and pick up a pack of sandwich crackers or pretzels and a diet soda. Is an 8- or 16-oz carton of skim milk or a container of yogurt available? The answer is yes. But, those are not the foods that come to mind in a convenience store. Is milk or yogurt available in your work cafeteria or local lunch spot? The answer again is yes. It is time to get your brain off of automatic pilot and to question your food choices.

Calcium: How much and where?

Most adults need 1000 mg of calcium per day. From ages 11–24, males and females need 1200–1500 mg each day. This is also the amount of calcium needed during pregnancy and breast feeding. Women not on estrogen replacement therapy and men over 65 should get 1500 mg a day. The best food sources of calcium are dairy products—milk, yogurt, and cheese—and dark green leafy vegetables such as broccoli, kale, and collards. (See page 161.) Also note that the sample meal plan on page 18 contains almost 1400 mg of calcium, mainly from milk, yogurt, light ice cream, cheese, and spinach.

Calcium beyond foods

Many physicians and RDs believe that adults, especially women of child-bearing years and post-menopausal women, should have more than 1000 mg of calcium each day. It is best to get calcium from foods; however, if you do not eat enough calcium, discuss a supplement with your health-care provider. Perhaps a 500- or 600-mg calcium tablet combined with at least 1 or 2 servings of milk or yogurt can help you reach the 1000 mg you need. Most multivitamin and mineral supplements contain very little calcium. Some health-care providers suggest that you use a calcium-containing antacid as your calcium supplement.

For people with lactose intolerance who avoid dairy products, a calcium supplement is especially important. You can purchase lactose-free milk. You can buy a product to add to milk and other lactose-containing foods called Lactaid. Lactaid breaks down lactose so that you can eat dairy foods without problems. Try to eat vegetables and fruits that contain calcium, too.

Calcium, milk, and osteoporosis

You need calcium throughout your life. Osteoporosis is a breaking down of the bones that leaves bones thinner, more brittle, and at risk of fractures. Anyone can get osteoporosis. However, women, especially smaller women with less bone mass, are at greater risk. Another reason more women develop osteoporosis today is that we live longer, and a decrease in the female hormone estrogen after menopause can add to loss of bone mass. One reason your doctor might recommend estrogen replacement therapy is to prevent osteoporosis.

To help prevent osteoporosis, eat enough calcium; walk, jog, dance, or ride a bike five days a week; and lift weights once or twice a week. Weight-bearing exercise keeps you from losing bone.

Milk and diabetes

People with diabetes are at the same risk for osteoporosis. Eating nonfat and low-fat milk and yogurt will give you the calcium you need without saturated fat and cholesterol.

Actually, as a person with diabetes, you may have an easier time fitting in 2 or 3 milk servings a day if you need to eat one or more snacks. Use a serving of milk or yogurt as a snack or part of a snack—milk and crackers or yogurt and fruit. Also, you might find that nonfat milk or yogurt makes a good food to treat low blood glucose reactions. They both provide as much carbohydrate as a serving of starch or fruit.

How many servings

Two to three servings a day. The chart below gives the specific number of servings to eat based on your calorie range.

	For weight loss for some women	Many older women	Many women, older adults	Older men, larger women	Kids, teen girls, active women, most men	Teen boys, active men
Calorie level	1200	1400	1600	1800	2200	2800
Servings*	2	2	2–3	2–3	2–3	2–3

*Teenagers, young adults to age 24 years, and women who are pregnant or breastfeeding need 1200–1500 mg of calcium each day. That equals about 4 servings of milk and yogurt. Use nonfat milk and yogurt to keep fat grams and calories low.

Look at this sample 1-day food plan to see how easy it is to have 2 servings of milk and yogurt (in **bold** type). Nutrient information is on page 18.

Breakfast
   1 whole oat bran English muffin
   1/2 large grapefruit
   2 Tbsp light cream cheese

Lunch
   1 pita pocket, 6" across, cut in half to fill
   1/3 medium sliced tomato
   1/3 cup sliced cucumbers

1/2 cup sliced large carrots or whole baby carrots
1 oz lean ham or turkey
1 oz part-skim Swiss cheese
Mustard to spread on bread
1 cup of low-fat/skim milk (1 serving)

Afternoon Snack

1 cup nonfat fruited yogurt sweetened with low-calorie sweetener (1 serving)
2 small tangerines

Dinner

5 oz dry red wine
1 cup spaghetti
1 whole wheat dinner roll
1 cup tomato sauce made with
    3/4 cup prepared tomato sauce
    1/3 cup onions
    1/3 cup peppers
    2 tsp canola oil (use to sauté onions and peppers)
    2 oz ground turkey, browned and drained (3 oz raw)
Spinach salad with
    1 cup spinach
    1/3 cup sliced mushrooms
    1 tsp purple onion
    2 Tbsp reduced-fat French salad dressing

Evening Snack

1/2 cup light ice cream
1 1/4 cups whole strawberries, sliced

A serving of milk

A serving is: 1 cup of milk or yogurt. Each serving of skim or non-fat milk or yogurt is 12 g of carbohydrates, 8 g of protein, no fat, and 90 calories. This is the same as a milk exchange. Once you start adding fat, as in low-fat milk or yogurt, the fat grams and calories climb. Remember, how important it is to eat correct serving sizes. At home, you can mark a glass so you know where the 1-cup line is. Otherwise, measure on occasion to make sure you're estimating correctly. Yogurt is easier with 6- or 8-oz containers. If you purchase larger containers or need to eat smaller amounts, measure the serving.

Nutrition assets

Milk and yogurt are a nice package of carbohydrate and protein. You may not often think of milk and yogurt as good sources of carbohydrate, but 1 serving contains almost as much as a serving of starch. Milk and yogurt do poorly in the fiber department but are excellent sources of many vitamins and minerals. You know about their superior calcium content. In addition, milk and yogurt are good sources of riboflavin, magnesium, phosphorus, and potassium. Because most milk today is fortified with vitamin D, milk is also a good source of this fat-soluble vitamin. For more about vitamins and minerals, see pages 158–162.

Lean on low-fat milk

Regular milk has between 3 and 4% fat. You will find several low-fat milks, some are 2% fat (about 5 g of fat per cup), others are 1% fat (about 3 g of fat per cup). And, nonfat or skim milk has 0% fat. A cup of whole milk has almost double the calories that skim milk has. All those calories are from fat, and some of it is saturated. Also, because milk is an animal product, it contains some cholesterol. If you choose skim milk, you drop the cholesterol per cup from 33 mg in whole milk to 4 mg in skim milk. So, choosing nonfat drops the undesirables—total fat and cholesterol—and still gives you all the great nutrition. The same goes for yogurt.

Get to know yourself

If you want to change your eating habits, you need to learn what you eat now. Ask yourself these questions:

▲ How many servings of milk or yogurt do I consume each day?

▲ Do I measure out my portions of milk?

▲ What type (percent fat) of milk and refrigerated and frozen yogurt do I buy?

▲ Do I add milk or yogurt to foods when eating or cooking—for example, milk to prepare hot cereal or top fruit with frozen yogurt?

▲ Am I between 11 and 24 years of age, pregnant, or breastfeeding? If yes, do I know I have a calcium requirement of 1200–1500 mg per day?

Change...one step at a time

Using your answers to the above questions, set your goals to change one step at a time. How many servings of milk or yogurt should you eat each day to meet your calcium requirement? If you don't drink any, explore how you can fit in one serving a day. Perhaps a cup of fruited yogurt would make a good afternoon snack, or you can substitute low-fat milk for diet soda at your employee cafeteria. If you know your calcium intake is shy of your needs, talk to your doctor or dietitian about a calcium supplement. Remember, a multivitamin and mineral supplement does not have much calcium.

Easy ways to get more milk and yogurt

▲ Eat more hot cereal, using milk to substitute for at least half (if not all) the water to cook the cereal, use more milk on the cereal as you eat it.

▲ Eat more high-fiber dry cereal, it is a way to consume more milk and get a good boost of fiber.

▲ Don't limit cereal and milk to breakfast; it can be a quick and easy lunch, dinner, or snack. It is a great way to work in another fruit serving, too.

▲ Blend a milk or yogurt shake for a tasty snack: put a serving of milk or yogurt in a blender, add a serving of fruit (banana, strawberries, or peach), add a bit of extract (vanilla, rum, or maple), blend it up, sip it down.

▲ Create your own yogurt combo. Take plain nonfat yogurt or frozen yogurt and toss in Grape-Nuts and/or low-fat granola cereal and dried fruit (diced dried apricots, apples, or pears), and add a few nuts for good crunch.

▲ Drop a few tablespoons of refrigerated yogurt on fresh or canned fruit.

▲ Use plain yogurt as a substitute for sour cream on potatoes. Mix in fresh herbs, garlic, dijon mustard, cayenne, or curry (or any combination of herbs and spices) for some extra kick.

▲ Make yogurt cheese the thickness of cream cheese and add some no-sugar jelly to spread on bagels or toast.

▲ Keep containers of yogurt in the refrigerator to use as a quick and convenient snack or part of a meal.

▲ Add dry milk to recipes where the taste will blend in—meat loaf or meatballs, soups, casseroles, gravies.

▲ Add skim milk or dry milk to eggs for scrambled eggs, omelettes, or French toast.

Now you know

▲ How many servings, on average, of milk and yogurt you consume daily.

▲ How many servings of milk and yogurt you should consume each day.

▲ Easy ways to get more milk and yogurt.

▲ The nutrition benefits of milk and yogurt.

▲ Steps to take if you know you will not get enough calcium from foods.

Scenario

Meet Dorothy. She is 33 years old, is 28 weeks pregnant with her second child, and just found out she has gestational diabetes (diabetes that occurs only during pregnancy). Dorothy's first child was 9.3 pounds at birth, and the doctor suspects she had gestational diabetes toward the end of that pregnancy. Dorothy has gained about 20 pounds since the beginning of her first pregnancy and that is one reason why her blood glucose is higher at an earlier stage of pregnancy.

She and her doctors want to control her blood glucose with her meal plan as long as possible; however, it is likely she will need to go on insulin toward the end of the pregnancy. When Dorothy met with the dietitian after her diagnosis, they talked about what she eats, particularly how much milk and yogurt due to her higher calcium needs.

Dorothy said, she sometimes has a bowl of dry cereal with 2% milk, maybe a green leafy vegetable a few times a week, and a cup of low-fat frozen yogurt about four nights a week. Dorothy gets some additional calcium from a prenatal multivitamin and mineral tablet. The RD and Dorothy saw that she is not getting the 1200–1500 mg of calcium that she needs during pregnancy—she eats about half the amount of calcium she needs.

Dorothy and her RD developed some ways she could get more calcium. Instead of skipping breakfast, she could have a creamy fruit shake, a breakfast drink, a can of a nutrition drink, or supplement designed for people with diabetes. Each provides about as much calcium as a cup of milk as well as other nutrients.

The RD encouraged Dorothy to eat breakfast before she leaves for work. Dry or cooked cereal with skim milk is a great choice. She should make cooked cereal with skim milk, not water, and then use more milk on the cooked cereal. Another quick breakfast that offers calcium is cheese toast (melted cheese on bread). For snacks, the dietitian suggested crackers and cheese (low fat or reduced calorie), a nonfat fruited yogurt, frozen yogurt with fresh fruit, custard, or pudding. The RD gave her quick and easy recipes for custard and pudding, and suggested she buy sugar-free, ready-to-eat containers or packaged mix. For a portion of frozen yogurt, the RD recommended a 1/2 cup serving instead of 1 cup.

These suggestions alone will not get Dorothy's calcium up to 1200–1500 mg each day. The dietitian suggested that she take another 600 mg a day of calcium as a supplement. She needs to call her physician to discuss this, because there is some calcium in the prenatal vitamins that she is taking.

Last, the RD encouraged Dorothy to schedule several follow-up visits during her pregnancy and to return after her baby is born. If Dorothy is going to breastfeed, her nutritional needs will be nearly the same as for pregnancy. When she is finished breastfeeding, she can begin to work on losing some weight. The dietitian noted that about 40% of women who have diabetes during pregnancy develop type II diabetes later in life. She encouraged Dorothy to listen to the warning sign of gestational diabetes. Dorothy could reduce her chances of developing diabetes if she keeps her weight controlled and walks or exercises regularly. Because she is at risk for diabetes, she should have her blood glucose checked once a year.

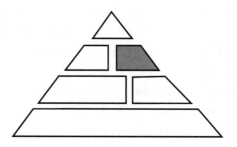

CHAPTER 7

MEAT GOES ON THE SIDE

What you will learn

▲ The number of servings of meat and other protein foods you should eat each day.

▲ The definition of a meat serving and the best ways to measure these foods.

▲ Easy ways to eat smaller amounts of protein foods.

▲ Easy ways to select and prepare meats and other protein foods in low-fat ways.

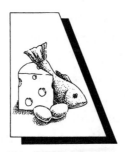

Meat and others near the top

Meat and others (protein foods) are next to the milk section and the same size. So, what is the pyramid's message about meat and others? You should have 2 or 3 servings per day of 2- to 3-oz portions. That means a total of no more than 5–7 oz a day. Many people eat that amount (or more) in one dinner.

Meats and other protein foods provide necessary protein and nutrients, but many animal protein foods (such as beef, chicken, and cheese) carry unhealthy partners—saturated fat and cholesterol. The whopping dose of fat quickly runs the calories up. Your goal is to eat meat as a side dish (a small portion), rather than letting it have the center of the plate. Remember to give the middle of the plate to starches and vegetables.

The meat and others group

What is in the meat and others group? Foods that are a good source of protein. Most are foods from an animal and are complete sources of protein. Complete protein means they contain the eight essential amino acids in the correct proportion—what you need to build muscle and body parts.

In the Diabetes Food Pyramid the word *meat* does not refer only to beef. It includes lamb; pork; veal; poultry including chicken, turkey, and duck; all seafood, including fish and shellfish. The "others" are cheese, including hard and soft cheeses and cottage cheese; eggs; and peanut butter.

America's report card on meats

Americans eat too much protein. Protein captures the spotlight at meals. Historically, this has been the way to show wealth, by dining on large servings of meat. Many Americans will chow down on a three-egg omelette with cheese for breakfast and then have 8–10 oz of rib eye steak or three pieces of chicken for dinner. But we would be wiser to try some dishes from other countries, where a small amount of protein is mixed with grains and vegetables to go a long way. Too much of the protein we eat is from animal sources—too much fat, saturated fat, and cholesterol. It is time to put meats in their place—near the top of the pyramid and on the side of the plate.

Hooray for vegetarianism

Picture your plate—small amounts of protein surrounded by plenty of vegetables, starches, and fruits. That is healthy eating. Vegetarians are a step ahead of the rest of us. Because meats are the best sources of certain nutrients, such as iron and zinc, a vegetarian needs to know how to get all the necessary vitamins and minerals from other foods. This is difficult if a vegetarian chooses to avoid milk or egg products as well as meats. There is protein in grains and beans, but to learn how to balance vegetarian meals, talk to your dietitian.

Protein and diabetes

People with diabetes have no less or more need for protein than the general public. The guideline suggests eating between 10 and 20% of your calories as protein. Extra protein works your kidneys harder to get rid of protein waste products. According to new research, people with diabetes may be healthier if they eat more of their protein from nonanimal sources (vegetables, beans, and grains).

Another reason to eat less animal protein is to get less fat and cholesterol. People with diabetes have a greater risk of heart disease earlier in life. One of the strongest guidelines is to eat less saturated fat. A quick way to do that is to cut down on animal protein foods—meats and whole milk dairy foods. If you cut down on animal protein, you can be pretty sure you will cut down on fat and cholesterol as well.

How many servings

Two to three servings a day. The chart on the next page gives you some suggestions for the number of servings or ounces of meat and others to eat based on your calorie range.

	For weight loss for some women	Many older women	Many women, older adults	Older men, larger women	Kids, teen girls, active women, most men	Teen boys, active men
Calorie level	1200	1400	1600	1800	2200	2800
Servings/Oz	2/4	2/4	2/5	2/5	2/6	2–3/7

Look at this sample 1-day food plan to see how to keep servings from the meat and other group to 2 servings or 6 oz. The nutrient information for this menu is on page 18. The meat servings are in **bold** so you can count them.

Breakfast
1 whole oat bran English muffin
1/2 large grapefruit
2 Tbsp light cream cheese

Lunch
1 pita pocket, 6" across, cut in half to fill
1/3 medium sliced tomato
1/3 cup sliced cucumbers
1/2 cup sliced large carrots or whole baby carrots
1 oz lean ham or turkey (1/2 serving)
1 oz part-skim Swiss cheese (1/2 serving)
Mustard to spread on bread
1 cup of low-fat/skim milk

Afternoon Snack
1 cup nonfat fruited yogurt sweetened with low-calorie sweetener
2 small tangerines

Dinner
> 5 oz dry red wine
> 1 cup spaghetti
> 1 whole wheat dinner roll
> 1 cup tomato sauce made with
>> 3/4 cup prepared tomato sauce
>> 1/3 cup onions
>> 1/3 cup peppers
>> 2 tsp canola oil (use to sauté onions and peppers)
>> **2 oz ground turkey, browned and drained (3 oz raw)**
>> **(1 serving)**
> Spinach salad with
>> 1 cup spinach
>> 1/3 cup sliced mushrooms
>> 1 tsp purple onion
>> 2 Tbsp reduced-fat French salad dressing

Evening Snack
> 1/2 cup light ice cream
> 1 1/4 cups whole strawberries, sliced

A serving of meat

The chart at the end of this chapter shows the serving sizes for foods in the meat and others group with each food's calorie, fat, saturated fat, and cholesterol content. A serving of most of the foods in the group is 2–3 oz, cooked. Here are some quick rules to translate from raw to cooked servings:

▲ Raw meat with no bone: 4 oz raw is 3 oz cooked
▲ Raw meat with bone: 5 oz raw is 3 oz cooked
▲ Raw poultry with skin: skin is 1/4–1/2 oz per 4–5 oz raw (remove skin before cooking or before serving)

You count some of the foods by the ounce, such as one egg or 2 Tbsp of peanut butter. If you use exchanges, be aware that 1 pyramid serving of meat is 3 oz and an exchange serving of meat is 1 oz.

(Although the serving sizes are different, both systems encourage you to eat the same amount of protein foods.)

An ounce of meat has about 7 g of protein, no matter what kind of meat it is. What makes the difference is the amount of fat. Very lean meats, such as white meat chicken or flounder have 0–3 g of fat and 70–105 calories per serving. Lean meat, such as sirloin or flank steak or dark meat chicken, has more fat, 6–9 g and 110–165 calories per serving. Medium-fat meat, such as ground beef or pork chops, has even more fat, 10–15 g and 150–225 calories per serving. High-fat meat, such as country pork ribs and regular cheese, has the most fat, 16–24 g of fat and 200–300 calories per serving.

Weigh and measure

It is important to weigh protein foods on occasion. It is easy to keep inching up when you cut off a wedge of cheese or guess the weight of a pork chop. In a restaurant, you can eyeball a correct serving as about the size of a deck of cards or a mayonnaise jar lid.

Which meat is leanest?

The fact is that fat content is decided by the cut of meat, not whether it is beef, lamb, pork, or veal. You can buy lean cuts of any meat. For the most part, chicken or turkey without the skin is leaner than most red meat. Also, most fish and shellfish are leaner than red meat.

A note of caution about organ meats—they are low in fat but quite high in cholesterol, especially liver. Remember, variety is the spice of life and also the way you get a balance of vitamins and minerals. So, bottom line, consider the fat and saturated fat grams, but also remember to eat what you enjoy and enjoy what you eat.

Ready to cook

Whether a selection of meat is still low fat when it gets to the table depends on how you cook it. To keep fat on the light side, limit deep-frying and don't use a lot of oil, butter, or cream sauces. Try low-fat cooking methods and try the sauces and seasonings suggested on page 71.

Stay lean and low fat

Many protein foods do not get cooked—cheese, canned tuna, or cold cuts. Many of these foods come in lean and low-fat varieties. You can choose from fat-free and low-fat cottage cheese, reduced-calorie cheese, water-packed tuna, lean cold cuts, and lean hot dogs. (Check the chart on pages 75–82.) Before you drop them in your supermarket cart, read the food label.

Downsize meat portion sizes

If your usual portion of meat, whether ham in a sandwich or several lamb chops, has typically been upward of 6, 8, or 10 oz, then 3 oz will seem tiny. To have long-term success, you need to downsize slowly, 1 oz at a time. If you usually eat 5–6 oz of turkey in a sandwich, step down to 4 oz, then to 3 oz month by month. Stuff sandwiches with lettuce, tomato, sliced cucumber, and sprouts. When you downsize servings, weigh items more frequently to help your eye adjust. Even if your servings are a bit larger than desirable in the beginning, choosing lean cuts and preparing food in low-fat ways are moves in a healthy direction.

Nutrition assets

In general, protein foods take longer to digest, in part because they are high in fat. That's why you feel full longer. Some are good sources of iron, zinc, vitamin B_6, B_{12}, thiamin, riboflavin, niacin, and phosphorus. (To learn more about vitamins and minerals, see pages 158–162.)

Get to know yourself

If you want to change your eating habits, you need to know what you're eating now. Ask yourself these questions and write down the answers:

▲ How many times a day do I eat meat and other protein foods?
▲ Do I believe I need to eat a food from the meat and others group at every meal?

▲ How many ounces of meat and other protein foods do I eat each day?

▲ What cuts of meat do I buy—are they higher fat or lower fat?

▲ What is my typical portion of meat or other protein food at breakfast, lunch, dinner, and snacks at home, at restaurants (fast food and upscale)?

▲ Do I weigh portions of protein foods?

▲ Do I buy lower-fat and fat-free meat and other protein foods?

▲ What cooking methods do I use for meat and other protein foods?

▲ What sauces and seasonings do I use on meat and other protein foods?

Change...one step at a time

Use your answers to the above questions to set your goals for healthy eating. How many ounces of protein do you need to eat each day? If your portions are now double what you need, think of ways to cut down. Collect a group of easy recipes that use just a smidgeon of meat—salad topped with marinated flank steak or tomato sauce with low-fat turkey sausage. Can you have a non-meat meal twice a week—vegetarian lasagna, bean burritos, black bean soup? Can you split an entree in a restaurant and order extra starches and vegetables—half a 10-oz steak, baked potato, and a trip to the salad bar? Start to think of meat as the side dish and not the center of the meal. If you currently eat meats fried or in heavy cream or butter sauces, try some new cooking methods and flavors.

Easy ways to slice off meat and others

▲ Split sandwiches in restaurants and ask for extra pieces of bread or roll. Share a salad plate, for example tuna or chicken salad, and request bread or rolls on the side. Make your own sandwiches with less protein and more vegetables.

▲ Make room on your plate for grains, starches, and vegetables, and only leave a little room on the side for meat.

- ▲ Buy smaller quantities (just what you need for the recipe) so you eat less.
- ▲ Cook dishes that s-t-r-e-t-c-h protein.
- ▲ Load sandwiches with raw vegetables (easier with pita bread because you can stuff the pocket).
- ▲ In fast-food restaurants, order single, regular, or junior-size sandwiches and stay away from the doubles and triples.
- ▲ Start the day without a serving of meat at breakfast: try a bowl of cereal, a bagel, or an English muffin.
- ▲ Gather recipes that have only a little meat and lots of grains and vegetables. Try to make a new one each week or two.

Low-fat cooking techniques, sauces, and seasonings

- ▲ Grill with different flavored wood chips—mesquite, hickory.
- ▲ Barbecue with barbecue sauce.
- ▲ Poach in broth, garlic, herbs, wine, sherry, or any combination of flavors.
- ▲ Marinate meat, chicken, or fish for several hours in fat-free ingredients before cooking. For starters: sherry, mustard, and garlic; soy or teriyaki sauce; ginger and garlic; vinegar (any variety); or garlic and basil.
- ▲ Make low-fat gravy using the drippings but little of the fat. Refrigerate the drippings until the fat turns solid and floats on top. Remove the fat. (Put drippings in a pan, add a bit of flour or cornstarch with a whisk, heat to thicken.) Puree any celery, onion, carrots, that were in the roasting pan and add to defatted gravy mixture to thicken.
- ▲ Use salsa or pico de gallo to spice up ground beef, chicken, or shrimp for fajitas, burritos, or soft tacos.
- ▲ Mix plain low-fat yogurt with mustard and dill to top fish.
- ▲ Make low-fat tartar sauce with low-fat or fat-free mayonnaise and relish.

Now you know

▲ To eat less meat and other protein foods each day.

▲ The nutrition assets and liabilities of meat and other protein foods.

▲ How to choose lower-fat cuts of meat and lower-fat varieties of other protein foods.

▲ How to s-t-r-e-t-c-h protein to eat small amounts.

▲ How to prepare meats and other protein foods with less fat.

Scenario

Meet Jocquin. He is 68 years old and works as a technician for a local cable television company. He is very inactive at his job. Jocquin has had type II diabetes for about 18 years. It was his 50th birthday present. He has not taken great care of his diabetes, partly because he never felt bad with high blood glucose.

Now, however, he is suffering the consequences. Jocquin just found out he has some initial signs of diabetes kidney disease, a small amount of protein in his urine (microalbuminuria). Jocquin's doctor advised him to speak with a dietitian about making some changes in what he eats to get his blood glucose in control and help delay further kidney damage. Jocquin was concerned and quickly made an appointment with the dietitian at a local diabetes program.

The RD started by asking Jocquin what he usually eats. She asked him be as honest as possible. She quickly found that Jocquin eats a lot of meat. Jocquin typically eats 2 large servings of meat each day. Lunch is often a large Italian submarine sandwich, a double cheeseburger, or a mile-high corned beef sandwich from a local sandwich shop. Dinner is often upward of 6 oz of chicken breast, hamburger, pork chops, or several pieces of fried fish.

Because Jocquin eats a lot of protein and he has the beginning signs of kidney disease, the dietitian decided to focus her teaching and suggestions on protein. First, the RD told him that he eats much more protein than his body needs. She added that better control of blood glucose can slow kidney damage, too. The dietitian gave Jocquin a few suggestions for cutting back on the amount of protein he eats.

Some lunch ideas:

▲ In a sub shop, order a small sub with turkey, smoked turkey, or roast beef. Hold the mayonnaise and oil and ask for mustard and plenty of lettuce, tomatoes, and onions.

▲ In a fast-food spot, order a single hamburger or grilled chicken sandwich and fill up on baked potato or garden salad with a small amount of light dressing.

For dinner, she suggested that he purchase a small food scale so he can see how much he is eating. She suggested he try to eat no more than 5–6 oz of meat at dinner. He could make pasta, potatoes, rice, and other starches a bigger part of his dinner meal. He should try to get at least two vegetables or a double serving of one at dinner as well. As he learns what 5–6 oz looks like on a food scale and on his plate, he can eyeball the quantity he should eat when he is out for dinner and take home the extra. She suggested that he separate the portion he will eat from the one he will take home before starting to eat.

When he feels comfortable limiting the meat at dinner to 5–6 oz, he can drop down to 4–5 oz. His long-term goal is no more than two 2- to 3-oz servings of meat each day. That comes as a shock to Jocquin. Before he left, Jocquin made an appointment to return in about 3 weeks. At that time, he will bring his blood glucose record book with a list of the meals and snacks that he has eaten. They will discuss how he can improve glucose control and how he is doing with the new ways to eat less protein.

	Serving	Cal.	Protein (g)	Total Fat (g)	Sat. Fat (g)	Chol. (mg)
Beef						
Brisket, braised	1 oz	63	9	3	1	27
Chuck/blade pot roast	1 oz	62	9	2	1	29
Corned beef brisket	1 oz	72	5	5	2	28
Cubed steak	1 oz	58	9	2	1	27
Flank steak, broiled, lean	1 oz	59	8	3	1	19
Ground beef, broiled, extra lean	1 oz	73	7	5	2	24
Ground beef, broiled, lean	1 oz	78	7	5	2	25
Ground beef, broiled, regular	1 oz	82	7	6	2	26
Ground round	1 oz	56	10	1	1	26
Meat loaf	1 oz	57	5	4	3	26
Prime rib, roasted	1 oz	83	8	6	2	23
Rib roast, roasted	1 oz	65	8	4	1	23
Round steak, broiled	1 oz	55	8	2	1	23
Rump roast, braised	1 oz	60	9	2	1	27
Short ribs	1 oz	83	9	5	2	26
Sirloin	1 oz	54	9	2	1	25
Steak, porterhouse	1 oz	62	8	3	1	23
Steak, rib eye	1 oz	64	8	3	1	23
Steak, T-bone	1 oz	61	8	3	1	23
Stew meat	1 oz	66	9	3	1	28
Tenderloin, broiled	1 oz	67	8	4	1	24
Cheese						
American, processed (high sodium)	1 oz	106	6	9	6	27
American, low fat	1 oz	50	7	2	1	10
Blue	1 oz	100	6	8	5	23

	Serving	Cal.	Protein (g)	Total Fat (g)	Sat. Fat (g)	Chol. (mg)
Brie	1 oz	91	6	8	5	28
Cheddar/colby, low fat	1 oz	49	7	2	1	6
Cheddar	1 oz	114	7	9	6	30
Cottage cheese, nonfat	1/4 cup	35	7	0	0	5
low fat, 2%	1/4 cup	50	8	1	1	5
Cottage cheese, 4%	2 Tbsp	46	4	3	2	8
Cottage cheese, dry	1/4 cup	31	6	0	0	2
Fat-free cheeses	1 oz	37	6	0	0	0
Feta	1 oz	74	4	6	4	25
Gouda	1 oz	100	7	8	5	30
Gruyere	1 oz	116	8	9	5	31
Monterey Jack	1 oz	106	7	9	5	27
Mozzarella, light	1 oz	65	8	3	2	15
Mozzarella, part skim milk	1 oz	72	7	5	3	16
Parmesan, grated	2 Tbsp	46	4	3	2	8
Parmesan, grated, fat free	2 Tbsp	60	6	0	0	0
Provolone	1 oz	100	7	8	5	20
Ricotta, part skim milk	1/4 cup	86	7	5	3	19
Romano, grated	2 Tbsp	46	4	4	2	12
Roquefort	1 oz	100	6	8	5	23
Sticks/string	1 oz	78	8	5	3	15
Swiss	1 oz	107	8	8	5	26
Eggs						
Fresh, large	1	74	6	5	2	213
Substitute	1/4 cup	35	7	0	0	0
Whites	2	34	7	0	0	0
Yolk	1	59	3	0	0	213

	Serving	Cal.	Protein (g)	Total Fat (g)	Sat. Fat (g)	Chol. (mg)
Fish						
Anchovy	1 oz	37	6	1	0	17
Calamari	1 oz	30	5	0	0	75
Catfish, fillet	1 oz	43	5	2	1	18
Cod	1 oz	30	7	0	0	16
Flounder	1 oz	33	7	0	0	19
Fried, cornmeal coated	1 oz	65	5	1	1	23
Gefilte fish	1 oz	35	3	3	1	15
Grouper	1 oz	42	6	2	0	14
Haddock	1 oz	32	7	0	0	21
Halibut	1 oz	40	8	1	0	12
Herring, smoked	1 oz	62	7	4	1	23
Mackerel	1 oz	75	6	5	1	23
Mahi Mahi	1 oz	71	7	5	2	18
Perch	1 oz	37	6	1	0	29
Salmon, canned, water pack, drained	1 oz	40	6	2	0	11
Salmon, fillet, broiled/baked	1 oz	61	8	3	1	25
Sardines, oil pack, drained	2	50	6	3	0	34
Scrod	1 oz	36	6	1	0	19
Snapper	1 oz	54	7	3	1	19
Sole	1 oz	32	7	0	0	17
Swordfish	1 oz	50	7	2	1	13
Trout	1 oz	54	8	2	0	21
Tuna	1 oz	52	9	2	1	14
Tuna, canned, water pack, drained	1 oz	33	7	0	0	9
Tuna, canned, oil pack, drained	1 oz	56	8	2	0	5

	Serving	Cal.	Protein (g)	Total Fat (g)	Sat. Fat (g)	Chol. (mg)
Game						
Buffalo	1 oz	40	8	1	0	23
Duck, roasted	1 oz	57	7	3	1	25
Goose, roasted	1 oz	68	8	4	1	27
Pheasant, no skin	1 oz	38	7	1	0	19
Quail	1 oz	53	6	3	1	20
Rabbit	1 oz	58	9	2	1	24
Venison	1 oz	45	9	1	0	32
Lamb						
Ground lamb	1 oz	80	7	6	2	28
Leg, sirloin, roast, lean	1 oz	58	8	3	1	26
Loin roast/chop, roasted	1 oz	57	8	1	1	25
Rib, roast	1 oz	67	8	4	1	26
Organ meats						
Heart, beef, simmered	1 oz	50	8	2	1	55
Kidney, beef, simmered	1 oz	41	7	1	0	110
Liver, beef, braised	1 oz	46	7	1	1	110
Liver, chicken, simmered	1 oz	45	7	2	1	180
Sweetbreads, beef, simmered	1 oz	45	3	4	1	582
Tongue, beef, simmered	1 oz	80	6	6	3	30
Pork						
Bacon, fried, drained, 20 slices/pound	3	105	5	9	3	15

For your convenience, we've also printed return instructions on the other side of this letter.

Thanks again for your recent order and Good Luck in our Prize Draw!

You can reach us by phone at 0161 278 8460, Monday - Friday, 9 a.m. - 5:30 p.m.

Cordially,

Robert H. Treller

Robert H. Treller, for
Publishers Clearing House

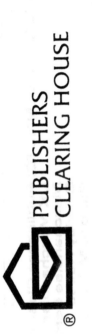

M7672UH

Dear Customer:

We really appreciate your business. I hope you'll be pleased with your purchase and continue to think of Publishers Clearing House as a fun, money saving place to shop.

We'd also like you to know that Publishers Clearing House stands behind every product we offer. If you should ever have a question or problem with an order -- at _any_ time --

	Serving	Cal.	Protein (g)	Total Fat (g)	Sat. Fat (g)	Chol. (mg)
Boston blade, roasted	1 oz	66	7	4	2	24
Canadian bacon, (high sodium)	1 oz	53	7	2	1	16
Chop, not loin	1 oz	73	7	4	1	20
Country-style ribs, lean only	1 oz	70	8	4	2	26
Cutlet, braised	1 oz	50	8	2	1	23
Ground pork	1 oz	84	7	6	2	27
Ham, boiled lean, sandwich type	1 oz	46	5	2	1	15
Ham, canned, fully cooked	1 oz	48	6	2	1	12
Ham, fresh, baked	1 oz	60	8	3	1	27
Ham, cured, roasted	1 oz	45	7	2	1	16
Loin, roast/chop, center cut roasted	1 oz	60	8	3	1	23
Sausage, fresh, patty/link, cooked	1 oz	105	6	9	3	24
Sausage, Italian, cooked	1 oz	92	6	7	3	22
Shoulder, blade/arm roast	1 oz	66	7	4	1	26
Spareribs, braised	1 oz	113	8	9	3	35
Tenderloin	1 oz	47	8	1	1	23

Poultry

	Serving	Cal.	Protein (g)	Total Fat (g)	Sat. Fat (g)	Chol. (mg)
Chicken, canned	1 oz	52	6	3	1	18
Chicken, dark meat, no skin	1 oz	58	8	3	1	26
Chicken, dark meat, with skin, roasted	1 oz	72	7	5	1	26
Chicken, fried, flour coated	1 oz	76	8	4	1	26

	Serving	Cal.	Protein (g)	Total Fat (g)	Sat. Fat (g)	Chol. (mg)
Chicken, white meat, with skin, roasted	1 oz	63	8	3	1	24
Chicken, white meat, no skin	1 oz	49	9	1	0	24
Cornish hen, no skin	1 oz	38	7	1	0	30
Ground turkey	1 oz	67	8	4	1	29
Turkey sausage	1 oz	65	5	5	2	46
Turkey, dark meat, no skin	1 oz	53	8	2	1	24
Turkey, white meat, no skin	1 oz	44	9	1	0	20

Processed meats

	Serving	Cal.	Protein (g)	Total Fat (g)	Sat. Fat (g)	Chol. (mg)
Bologna, beef and pork	1 oz	89	3	8	3	16
Bratwurst, pork, cooked	1 oz	85	4	7	3	17
Chipped beef (sodium)	1 oz	47	8	1	1	26
Hot dog, <1 g fat/oz (sodium)	1 oz	30	4	1	0	11
Hot dog, low-fat, <3 g fat/oz (sodium)	1	50	6	2	1	15
Hot dog, beef and pork, 10/pound, (sodium)	1	144	5	13	5	22
Hot dog, chicken, 10/pound, (sodium)	1	116	6	9	3	45
Hot dog, turkey, 10/pound, (sodium)	1	102	6	8	2	48
Kielbasa	1 oz	95	4	9	3	24
Knockwurst	1 oz	87	3	8	3	16
Liverwurst	1 oz	100	4	9	3	50

	Serving	Cal.	Protein (g)	Total Fat (g)	Sat. Fat (g)	Chol. (mg)
Pastrami, beef	1 oz	35	6	1	3	15
Pepperoni	1 oz	140	6	13	5	—
Pickle and pimiento loaf	1 oz	74	3	6	2	10
Salami, beef and pork	1 oz	71	4	6	2	18
Salami, turkey	1 oz	54	4	4	1	20
Sausage, <1 g fat/oz, hard	1 oz	35	5	1	0	12
Sausage, <5 g fat/oz	1 oz	45	4	3	1	15
Sausage, Polish	1 oz	92	4	8	3	20
Sausage, smoked	1 oz	96	4	9	3	20
Spam	1 oz	70	4	6	—	—
Turkey bacon	1 slice	35	2	2	1	10
Turkey ham, <1 g fat/oz	1 oz	36	5	1	1	16
Turkey kielbasa, <3 g fat/oz	1 oz	45	4	3	1	16
Turkey pastrami, <3 g fat/oz	1 oz	40	5	2	1	15
Vienna sausages	1 oz	69	3	7	2	15
Shellfish						
Clams, canned, drained, solids	1 oz	42	7	1	0	19
Clams, fresh, steamed	1 oz	42	7	1	0	19
Crab, canned, drained, solids	1 oz	28	6	0	0	26
Crab, steamed	1 oz	29	6	1	0	28
Imitation shellfish, from surimi	1 oz	29	3	0	0	6

	Serving	Cal.	Protein (g)	Total Fat (g)	Sat. Fat (g)	Chol. (mg)
Lobster, fresh, steamed	1 oz	28	6	0	0	20
Mussels	1 oz	48	7	1	0	16
Oysters, canned	1 oz	24	3	1	0	19
Oysters, fresh, medium, cooked	6	58	6	2	1	44
Scallops, fresh, steamed	1 oz	32	7	0	0	15
Shrimp, canned, drained, solids	1 oz	34	7	1	0	50
Shrimp, fresh, cooked in water	1 oz	28	6	0	0	56

Veal

	Serving	Cal.	Protein (g)	Total Fat (g)	Sat. Fat (g)	Chol. (mg)
Brisket, lean, roast	1 oz	47	7	2	1	31
Cutlet, lean, cooked	1 oz	58	11	2	1	38
Ground veal	1 oz	49	7	2	1	29
Loin/chop, cooked	1 oz	50	8	2	1	30

Others

	Serving	Cal.	Protein (g)	Total Fat (g)	Sat. Fat (g)	Chol. (mg)
Peanut butter, smooth, salted	1 Tbsp	188	8	16	3	0
Soy milk	1 cup	79	7	5	1	0
Tempeh	1/4 cup	83	8	3	1	0
Tofu	1/2 cup	88	9	6	1	0

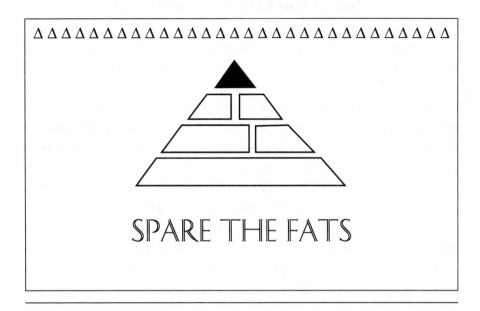

△ △

CHAPTER 8

SPARE THE FATS

What you will learn

▲ The total amount of fat you should eat each day.

▲ How the fat grams creep in and add up.

▲ How to eat fewer unhealthy fats (saturated fat).

▲ How to eat more of the "healthy" fats (monounsaturated fat).

▲ Easy ways to skim and spare the fats.

▲ Tips to slim down your favorite recipes.

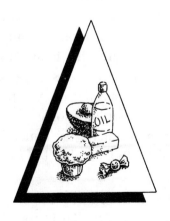

One of the three at the tip...fat

A threesome shares the tip of the pyramid—fats, sweets, and alcohol. These three take up the smallest space on the food pyramid, but we eat too much of them. That's why there's a chapter for each in this book.

What is the pyramid message about fats? Short and simple—eat less. That may be simple to say, but it's not simple to do, because fat is everywhere. It is in the obvious—butter and mayonnaise—and in the not so obvious—crackers, meat, cheese, and sweets. The pyramid gives no specific number of servings of fat to eat each day, but you do need a *little*. See page 90 to learn how to figure the grams of fat you need. To eat healthy you will also need to develop the skills of a detective—whether it is reading food labels in the supermarket or asking questions in restaurants—to detect fat grams wherever they hide.

What foods are fat

Some foods are almost 100% fat, such as butter, margarine, or regular salad dressing. Others contain a lot of fat, such as meats, cheese, nuts, whole milk dairy foods, and some desserts. But, plenty of foods contain no fat at all, such as pasta, broccoli, and apples.

So, what are the fats on the food pyramid? Fats are oils, butter, margarine, nuts, salad dressings, mayonnaise, and bacon—foods whose calories are mainly from fat. (Fat adds more calories per gram than any other type of food.)

Fats are divided into three types: saturated, polyunsaturated, and monounsaturated. Saturated fats come from animal foods (butter, whole milk, meats) and are the least healthy for your body. Polyunsaturated fats, such as corn or soybean oil, are a bit healthier. Monounsaturated fats, such as olive oil or canola oil, are the best fats you can eat. All foods with fat have some of each: saturated, polyunsaturated, and monounsaturated. Just remember that a little goes a long way. They are all 100% fat and full of calories.

America's report card on fats

We fail on fats. Whether it is the fat in french fries, a 10-oz prime rib, blue cheese dressing on salad, or a slice of apple pie a la mode, Americans love their fat. We are cutting back on the amount of fat we eat, but our calorie levels are going up! We fool ourselves when we choose low-fat or fat-free foods, thinking that these foods have no calories. They do—usually from added sugars.

Added and attached fats

To see how the fat grams creep into your meals divide them into two categories: added fats and attached fats. Added fats are fats that you put on and in foods. It is mayonnaise in seafood salad, cream cheese on bagels, sour cream on baked potatoes, and cream in a cream sauce or soup.

Attached fats are part of the food and can't let go. For example, there is no way to take the fat out of nuts, prime rib, or cheesecake. Fat is attached and there to stay.

Food with healthy fats

Let's get one thing straight about nuts, avocado, and olives, foods with so-called healthy fats. Their nutrients are surrounded by lots of fat grams and calories. All three are good examples of attached fats. They have been in the spotlight because some of their fat is the healthy monounsaturated fat variety. To decide how much of these foods to eat, check the number of calories you need, how important it is for you to increase your monounsaturated fats, and how well you can limit the amount of these foods that you eat. Nuts are especially difficult to stop eating when you've had just one serving.

Fat adds taste

Why is fat in so many foods? The answer is simple. Fat makes food taste good, and we like that flavor. Fats make you feel full. Fats also hold moisture in foods, such as baked goods and create the creamy texture of mayonnaise and salad dressings. Because fat plays so many roles in foods, it is difficult to make a great-tasting low-fat or fat-free food.

Fat calories add up

Along with flavor, fat adds calories. Nine calories per fat gram—twice as much as the 4 calories per gram for carbohydrate and protein. Fat comes in small, calorie-dense packages. That's one problem. The other is that fats from animal sources, whether butter, cheese, or chicken skin, add saturated fat and cholesterol. Consider how fat adds up in these examples:

Fat adds calories

Food	Serving	Calories	Fat (g)	Sat. fat (g)	Chol. (mg)
Bread	1 slice	65	1	0	0
Bread with 1 tsp butter	1 slice	100	5	2	10
Bread with 1 tsp margarine	1 slice	100	5	1	0
Macaroni	1 cup	197	1	0	0
Macaroni and cheese	1 cup	430	22	9	42
Chicken breast, roasted, no skin	3 oz	142	3	1	72
Chicken breast, roasted, with skin	3 oz	165	7	2	71
Chicken breast, fried, with skin	3 oz	218	11	3	71

Fats and diabetes

Fat ought to make up about 30% of your calories. The total amount of fat you eat should be based on the foods you like and your goals for blood glucose control. You need an individualized eating plan. For example, a young athlete with type I diabetes might need 4000 calories a day during football season. He probably needs 40% of his calories from fat just to get all those calories in. He still should choose foods with lower saturated fat and cholesterol and more monounsaturated fat.

The strongest guideline is to hold saturated fat to 10% of calories. Saturated fat raises blood cholesterol. High blood cholesterol is a risk factor for heart disease. People with diabetes have more frequent heart disease. Limiting saturated fat might help prevent that. Also, some people with blood lipid and triglyceride problems might benefit from increasing the amount of monounsaturated fats they eat. As for cholesterol, keep it to 300 mg each day.

How many servings?

You do not need to eat a specific number of fat servings. Just meet the grams or servings of fat in your meal plan. The chart below tells how many fat grams to eat if you want 20, 30, or 40% of your calories as total fat for different calorie ranges.

	For weight loss for some women	Many older women	Many women, older adults	Older men, larger women	Kids, teen girls, active women, most men	Teen boys, active men
Calorie level	1200	1400	1600	1800	2200	2800
Fat g for 20%	27	31	36	40	49	62
Fat g for 30%	40	47	53	60	73	93
Fat g for 40%	53	62	71	80	98	124

Page 90 tells how to calculate the amount of fat you should eat.

Look at the 1-day meal plan to see how to keep fats on the light side. There are 3 fat servings in **bold** type. There are 48 g of fat for the day (or 24% of the calories). The fat content is low for several reasons: low-fat choices are used, such as light cream cheese, nonfat yogurt, and light ice cream; mustard is used rather than mayonnaise; and the pasta is topped with a tomato sauce rather than a cream sauce. Ground turkey is used instead of ground beef, and it is browned and drained to remove some fat. The amount of monounsaturated fats is increased by using canola oil instead of corn oil to sauté the vegetables for the tomato sauce. These steps are in *italics* in the meal plan. See page 18 for nutrient information.

Breakfast
　　1 whole oat bran English muffin
　　1/2 large grapefruit
　　2 Tbsp light cream cheese (1 serving)

Lunch
　　1 pita pocket, 6" across, cut in half to fill
　　1/3 medium sliced tomato
　　1/3 cup sliced cucumbers
　　1/2 cup sliced large carrots or whole baby carrots
　　1 oz lean *ham or turkey*
　　1 oz *part-skim Swiss cheese*
　　Mustard to spread on bread
　　1 cup of *low-fat/skim milk*

Afternoon Snack
　　1 *cup nonfat fruited yogurt sweetened with low-calorie sweetener*
　　2 small tangerines

Dinner
　　5 oz dry red wine
　　1 cup spaghetti
　　1 whole wheat dinner roll
　　1 cup *tomato sauce* made with

3/4 cup prepared tomato sauce

1/3 cup onions

1/3 cup peppers

**2 tsp canola oil (use to sauté onions and peppers)
(2 servings)**

2 oz ground turkey, *browned and drained (3 oz raw)*

Spinach salad with

1 cup spinach

1/3 cup sliced mushrooms

1 tsp purple onion

2 Tbsp *reduced-fat French salad dressing*

Evening Snack

1/2 cup *light ice cream*

1 1/4 cups whole strawberries, sliced

A serving of fat

The chart at the end of the chapter shows the serving sizes for added fats along with information on their calorie, fat, and cholesterol content. Each fat serving has about 5 g of fat and 45 calories. The same as fat exchanges. Foods are divided by the fat they have the most of—saturated, polyunsaturated, and monounsaturated. All foods with fat have some of each of these types of fat. Because the calories from fat add up very quickly, it is particularly important to pay attention to serving sizes. An extra teaspoon of regular margarine is 50 calories. Measure fats from time to time to make sure your eyeballs are still estimating correctly.

Nutrition assets

You need a small amount of fat to carry the fat-soluble vitamins A, D, E, and K; to maintain healthy skin; and to become part of some hormones. But we can meet that need with a very small amount of fat, such as that you can get from chicken, cheese, crackers, and breads.

See pages 158–162 for more about the best foods to eat for certain vitamins and minerals.

How much fat to eat?

When it comes to fat, your first goal is probably going to be to eat less. When you lower the amount of fat, you automatically lower saturated fat and cholesterol. It is best to work with a dietitian to design a meal plan to fit the foods you like, your schedule, and your diabetes goals. For starters, here's how to figure the amount of fat to eat if 30% of your calories come from fat using a 2000-calorie meal plan.

Total number of calories: 2000 calories

To find 30 percent of 2000 calories,
multiply by 30% or .30:

$$2000 \text{ calories} \times .30$$
$$600 \text{ calories from fat}$$

There are 9 calories in a gram of fat. So to find how many *grams* of fat in 600 calories, divide by 9.

$$9\overline{)600} \quad 67 \text{ g of fat}$$

To figure how many grams of *saturated* fat to eat:
Multiply 2000 calories times 10% or .10
$2000 \times .10 = 200$ calories from saturated fat
(This is part of the 600 calories you figured above.)
Divide this number by 9. $200/9 = 22$ g of saturated fat
So, you can eat 67 g of fat for the day, and 22 g of that number can come from saturated fat.

Beyond total fat

All fats, whether butter, canola oil, or fat from meats, have different amounts of the three fatty acids—saturated, polyunsaturated, and monounsaturated. For example, butter is not all saturated fat and canola oil is not all monounsaturated fat. These fatty acids act differently on total blood cholesterol and LDL (the bad cholesterol) and HDL (the good cholesterol) as well as triglycerides. Here are the facts.

Saturated fats

Foods with saturated fat are mainly from animals. Red meats, poultry, seafood, whole milk, cheese, and butter all contain some saturated fat. Another group of foods—tropical oils such as coconut, palm, and palm kernel oil—are used in commercial foods such as crackers, cookies, and snack foods. How do you cut down on saturated fat? First, cut down on total fat. Then focus on decreasing the amount of animal products you eat.

▲ Meats—purchase lean cuts, cut off all visible fat before cooking, use preparation methods that get rid of more fat, such as grilling and measure your 2- to 3-oz servings (cooked).

▲ Poultry—take off the skin either before or after cooking and eat 2–3 oz servings (cooked).

▲ Seafood—choose lower-fat fish, prepare with small amounts of fat, and eat 2–3 oz servings (cooked).

▲ Cheese—limit amount you eat, buy part-skim, reduced-fat cheese.

▲ Butter—you can cut saturated fat in half by whipping 1 cup of canola oil with 1 cup of butter.

▲ Milk, yogurt—use the skim, nonfat, and fat-free varieties.

▲ Processed foods—check the labels for tropical oils or other fats. If they come at the end of the list, only small amounts of them were used in the food.

Look at the saturated fat content of the foods in the food lists of this and other chapters.

Polyunsaturated fats

On the positive side, polyunsaturated fats help lower blood cholesterol. On the negative, they lower good cholesterol (HDL) at the same time. About 10% of your fat calories should come from polyunsaturated fat. You find polyunsaturated fats mainly in liquid oils—corn, cottonseed, and soy. These oils are used in commercial crackers, cookies, and other foods. If you see "hydrogenated" oils on a food label, you may want to avoid those, because they are saturated.

Monounsaturated fats

Monounsaturated fats are known as the good guys. Monounsaturated fats offer the benefit of lowering cholesterol while not decreasing the body's good cholesterol (HDL). Research in people with type II diabetes shows that eating a diet high in monounsaturated fats and more moderate in carbohydrate (about 40%) can improve blood lipid levels. However, it is not easy to eat the amount of monounsaturated fats used in some studies. More research is needed, but here is advice about monounsaturated fats:

▲ Eat less total fat because that is the best way to control blood lipids. Do not eat more fat just to get monounsaturates.

▲ Stock canola and/or olive oil in your cupboard. Use to sauté, cook, bake (not olive oil to bake), and prepare salad dressings.

▲ Sprinkle a few nuts on foods, such as salads, desserts, or stir-fries.

▲ Use a slice or two of avocado on a salad, to garnish a casserole, for guacamole (a Mexican topping).

▲ Use a few olives on a relish plate, to toss in a salad, or as a garnish.

▲ Buy canola- or olive oil–based commercial salad dressings and canola-based margarine and mayonnaise, or make your own with canola or olive oil.

Cholesterol facts

Cholesterol is actually not fat. In fact, two foods that are very high in cholesterol are very low in fat—liver and shrimp. Another confusing point—foods high in saturated fat are not necessarily high in cholesterol or vice versa.

There is really no difference between the cholesterol content of lean meats and higher-fat meats. Cholesterol is discussed with fats because it is a fatlike substance that raises blood cholesterol.

The diabetes guidelines encourage you to eat no more than 300 mg of cholesterol daily. Dietary cholesterol is found, like saturated fat, in foods from animal sources—red meats, organ meats, poultry, seafood, egg yolk, and whole milk dairy foods. The leaders of the pack in terms of cholesterol content are liver, shrimp, calamari (squid), and egg yolk. You do not need to avoid these foods. Eat them in moderation.

Get to know yourself

If you want to change your eating habits, you need to know what you eat now. Ask yourself these questions:

▲ What added fats and how much of each do I use each day?

▲ What foods do I eat that provide attached fat?

▲ How much fat do I eat each day from attached fats?

▲ How often do I eat fried foods?

▲ What low-fat and fat-free foods do I enjoy and use to reduce fat?

▲ When I eat in restaurants, do I attempt to watch the fat grams?

Change...one step at a time

Use your answers to the above questions to take one step at a time toward healthy eating. How many grams of fat should you eat each day and how much saturated fat and cholesterol? If you found out that your fat consumption is sky high, then take a few steps to bring it down. Maybe you will eat fried foods one less time each week, order a small rather than large french fries at a fast-food restaurant, use fruit spread on toast rather than margarine, and so on.

Easy ways to spare and skim the fat

▲ Use skim (or no more than 1%) milk.

▲ Take advantage of light and reduced-fat cheese. Find out which products you like. Sometimes you can use less of the regular and still get the taste you enjoy.

▲ If a recipe calls for cheese and you want to use a regular type, buy a sharp variety, and use a smaller quantity. The sharper taste gives more flavor from a smaller amount.

▲ Try the low-fat, light, and fat-free products to see which taste OK to you. You might have to experiment—cream cheese, cottage cheese, mayonnaise, sour cream. Remember, these products are not calorie free. Be sure to read the Nutrition Facts.

▲ Buy the low-fat, reduced-calorie, or fat-free salad dressing that has the taste you like. No matter what salad dressing you use, pour it cautiously.

▲ Use plain nonfat yogurt or sour cream instead of regular products; add herbs and seasonings to make it tasty. Use it on baked potatoes, vegetables, chicken, and fish.

▲ Keep fresh lemon and lime on hand to squirt on vegetables and fish instead of more fat.

▲ When you buy meats, buy lean cuts; trim off excess fat; prepare in low-fat and moist ways.

▲ Marinate meats and vegetables in wine, vinegars, seasonings, and spices to add flavors without fat.

▲ Consider using applesauce, prune puree, or other dried fruit puree to replace fat in baked goods recipes. Check the back of boxes of these foods for some recipes or write to the manufacturer to request recipes.

Tips to slim down favorite recipes

What about Aunt Sally's macaroni and cheese recipe or Grandma Betty's apple cobbler? You long for them, but they are high in fat and calories from cheese, butter, and sugar. Well, learn to slim them down. Here are a few tips and guidelines:

▲ Think of a recipe as a starting point. Change it any way you want to make it tastier and healthier. For example, you might use less oil to sauté and add a few drizzles of cooking wine or sherry to add flavor without extra fat. Or maybe you raise the fiber of a meat loaf by adding bulgur, or increase the calcium in an omelette by adding a tablespoon of nonfat dry milk to the egg mixture.

▲ Keep in mind that it is easier to slim down recipes when you cook instead of bake. You cannot change recipes for some baked items such as chocolate cake or sponge cake because there is a delicate balance between ingredients. For example, if you cut the sugar in half or try to use a low-calorie sweetener (sugar substitute) in a chocolate cake, the result is a flatter and more dense cake. But, if you use less sugar or a low-calorie sweetener in a glaze to top chicken, the recipe turns out fine.

▲ You can change the recipes of some baked items. For instance, recipes that contain fruit, such as fruit cobbler, banana bread, or carrot or applesauce cake, will slim down. That is because the fruit provides both sweetness and bulk (volume) to the recipe. Or you can lower fat and calorie count of a pie by using a single bottom crust rather than top and bottom crusts. Look for a similar recipe in low-calorie or diabetes cookbooks. Adapt your recipe or try theirs.

▲ When you use less fat, you must add back flavor. For flavor add fat-free seasonings, spices, or herbs. Try new ones for new taste treats.

▲ Use more or less of an ingredient. For example, in a recipe for stir-fry use less meat (protein). Add volume with larger quantities of the vegetables in the recipe or add another vegetable, starch, or fruit. For instance, add pineapple chunks and bean sprouts. A few drops of spicy hot oil add flavor with few calories.

▲ In a meat sauce, use less meat and add more vegetables. For example, sauté onions, peppers, mushrooms, and zucchini to add volume to the tomato sauce. Or in a lasagna, use less meat and add a layer of spinach sautéed with a bit of oil and lots of garlic.

▲ Substitute an ingredient with more flavor so you can use less of it. Or take advantage of lean but flavorful sausage or textured vegetable protein (TVP) rather than a larger amount of ground meat in a chili or soup.

▲ Drain and pat dry ground meat or sausage to get out as much excess fat as you can.

▲ Sauté with less oil or butter than the recipe calls for. Just a reminder—you might need to use a lower flame than suggested to avoid burning the food.

▲ Use less sugar than a recipe calls for. You can usually use one-quarter to one-half less sugar. For example, stir-fry chicken and vegetables might call for 2 Tbsp of sugar. The recipe will taste as good with 1 tablespoon of sugar. Remember, you cannot make these changes as easily when you bake.

▲ Take advantage of new reduced-fat, reduced-calorie ingredients to use in some recipes. For example, top a Mexican dish with light or nonfat sour cream, make a dip with a combination of nonfat yogurt and light sour cream, or use light cream cheese to make a flavorful spread. A note of caution: be careful cooking or baking with these ingredients, such as margarinelike spreads listing water as the first ingredient. You put it in the pan to melt and what happens? The water separates from the oil and splatters on you. It is best to use these ingredients in noncooked recipes or as toppers after the item is cooked.

▲ Use fresh herbs. You can buy them in the supermarket. Buy them no more than a few days before you cook so they are fresh. If you do not use the fresh herb immediately, wrap it in a slightly damp paper towel and place it in a plastic bag. Use within a few days. The less expensive way to have herbs is to grow them. If your recipe calls for dried herbs, increase the amount of herb by three.

▲ Buy dry herbs and spices in small quantities because they lose taste over time. Clean out the cupboard every year. If you use dry herbs instead of fresh, use only one-third the amount.

▲ Check out recipe resources. Borrow low-calorie and diabetes cookbooks and magazines from the library. Purchase American Diabetes Association cookbooks, and order the monthly magazine *Diabetes Forecast*, which has timely new taste treats every month. Take advantage of healthy-cooking shows on television.

How to fine-tune your recipes

On the next page are some ingredients you can substitute in recipes to lower the fat and calories, lower the sugar, increase the healthiness, or increase flavor.

Now you know

▲ How fat sneaks in before you know it.
▲ That your body needs only a little bit of fat.
▲ Fat contributes lots of calories in a very small amount of food.
▲ What the three types of fat are.
▲ Many ways to spare the fat.
▲ Tips to slim down favorite recipes.

Ingredient	Substitution
Butter, regular stick	Margarine, regular stick or whip 1 cup oil and 1 cup butter to make your own soft butter
Cream cheese	Neufchatel, light, or fat free cream cheese
Mayonnaise	Reduced-calorie or fat-free mayonnaise or mix regular mayonnaise with nonfat yogurt
Meat, ground	Extra-lean ground meat or ground turkey
Milk, whole	Skim milk, 1% milk, or nonfat dry milk
Milk, evaporated	Evaporated skim milk
Nuts	Grape-Nuts, low-fat granola cereal, All Bran cereal
Oil for sautéing	Cooking wine and/or broth, cooking sprays
Sausage	Low-fat turkey sausage
Sour cream	Light or nonfat sour cream, nonfat plain yogurt, or low-fat cottage cheese, blenderized
Vegetable oil	Canola or olive oil (note: extra-virgin olive oil adds the most flavor)

Scenario

Meet Anna. Anna is 57 years old and works as an administrative assistant for an insurance company. She is Mexican-American. She recently found out that she has type II diabetes when she went to her doctor with symptoms of a yeast infection and blurred vision.

The diabetes did not come as a surprise, because many people in her family have it. Anna is overweight by about 30 pounds. For several years, she has had high blood pressure for which she takes medication and tries to watch her salt and sodium intake. When her doctor diagnosed diabetes, he also found her blood lipids were not normal. Her cholesterol was 265 (normal is less than 200), LDL was 186 (normal is less than 130), and HDL was 32 (normal is more than 35).

Anna's doctor suggested she try to control both her diabetes and blood lipids with changes in her eating habits and some weight loss before starting any diabetes medication. Her doctor gave her some pamphlets to read about what she should try to eat and how to find an RD.

Anna was anxious to see a dietitian because she just was not feeling herself. She went 1 week later. The RD told Anna that it is common for people with type II diabetes who are overweight to also have high blood pressure and blood lipids. She stressed how important it is to control these things to be healthy for many years. The best news Anna heard is that losing just a few pounds should improve all these problems.

Anna listed what she usually eats. For breakfast during the week, Anna has a large muffin with margarine or a bagel with cream cheese and coffee. Weekend breakfasts are doughnuts, a cinnamon bun, or a cheese omelette along with toast and jam.

She often eats lunch in the employee cafeteria—tuna or chicken salad sandwich with chips and coleslaw. Sometimes she has fried chicken, mashed potatoes, and gravy with a green vegetable. Other times she goes out for a few slices of pizza with extra cheese and pepperoni or a hamburger and large french fries and regular soda.

She eats dinner at home and often has chicken or fish—fried because that is how her husband likes it. She tries to eat one vegetable at dinner and adds margarine to that. That is her weakness. She has 2 or 3 slices of bread with margarine at dinner. In the evening she munches on cookies, chips, or ice cream.

The RD showed Anna the food pyramid so that she could see that she eats too much protein and fats and too few vegetables, fruits, and milk. The first area to work on was eating less fat. They developed a list of ways to lower fat, saturated fat, and cholesterol.

For breakfast Anna will bring a bagel from home and use light or fat-free cream cheese; if she has a muffin, she'll leave off the margarine. A breakfast of cereal, milk, and fruit at home would be great. The RD suggested Anna bring pieces of fruit to work to eat for breakfast, lunch, or a snack.

For lunch, Anna would be better off choosing a plain meat sandwich—turkey, roast beef, and sometimes ham—rather than tuna or chicken salad. She can request mustard rather than mayonnaise and get more lettuce and tomato on top. A bag of pretzels without salt, a small salad, or a cooked vegetable would be lower-fat side items. For hot meals, a vegetable plate, keeping fried items few and far between, would be healthy; as would a trip to the cafeteria salad bar, or roasted chicken with two vegetables. Pizza is fine as long as it is topped with vegetables rather than high-fat extra cheese and meats.

At dinner, Anna should roast, grill, steam, or poach chicken or fish rather than fry it. Again she should try to eat 2 servings of vegetables. Rather than margarine on top, the dietitian suggested a squirt of lemon juice or a dash of a low-sodium herb combination. She encouraged Anna to buy some great-tasting whole wheat bread and to try to enjoy it with no margarine or a light spread. For evening snacks, Anna could try nonfat, sugar-free yogurt with fruit, cereal and skim milk, light popcorn, or low-salt pretzels, watching how much sodium she gets. Anna was willing to try these suggestions and to come back in several weeks.

	Serving	Cal.	Total fat (g)	Sat. fat (g)	Mono. fat (g)	Poly. fat (g)	Chol. (mg)
Fats, monounsaturated							
Almonds, dry roasted, whole	6	47	4	0	3	1	0
Avocado, fresh	1/8	40	4	1	2	1	0
Cashews, oil roasted, whole	6	52	4	1	3	1	0
Macadamias, oil roasted, whole	3	46	5	1	4	0	0
Mixed nuts, <50% peanuts	6	37	3	1	2	1	0
Oils							
Canola	1 tsp	41	5	0	3	1	0
Olive	1 tsp	40	5	1	3	0	0
Peanut	1 tsp	40	5	1	2	1	0
Sesame	1 tsp	40	5	1	2	2	0
Olives, green, large, stuffed (high sodium)	10	50	4	0	2	—	0
Olives, ripe, large, pitted	8	40	4	1	3	0	0
Peanut butter, smooth, salted	2 tsp	63	5	1	3	2	0
Peanuts, dry roasted, no salt, all types	10	44	5	1	2	1	0
Peanuts, oil roasted, shelled	10	57	5	1	—	—	0
Peanuts, raw, shelled	10	54	5	1	2	1	0
Pecans, halves	4	46	5	0	3	1	0
Pine nuts, dried	1 Tbsp	40	4	1	2	2	0
Pistachio nuts, dry roasted, shelled	1 Tbsp	43	4	1	—	—	0
Sesame seeds	1 Tbsp	52	5	1	2	2	0
Tahini paste	2 tsp	59	5	1	2	2	0

	Serving	Cal.	Total fat (g)	Sat. fat (g)	Mono. fat (g)	Poly. fat (g)	Chol. (mg)
Fats, polyunsaturated							
Margarine, stick, >80% veg. oil	1 tsp	34	4	1	2	1	0
Margarine, tub, >75% veg. oil	1 tsp	30	4	1	0	1	0
Margarine, squeeze, >70% veg. oil	1 tsp	30	3	1	1	2	0
Margarine, lower fat, 30–50% veg. oil	1 Tbsp	50	6	1	2	2	0
Margarine, reduced calorie	1 Tbsp	50	6	1	3	2	0
Mayonnaise	1 tsp	33	4	1	1	2	3
Mayonnaise, light, reduced fat	1 Tbsp	40	3	1	1	3	6
Miracle Whip salad dressing, regular	2 tsp	39	3	1	1	2	3
Miracle Whip salad dressing, reduced calorie	1 Tbsp	45	4	1	1	2	5
Oils							
Corn	1 tsp	44	5	1	1	3	0
Safflower	1 tsp	44	5	1	1	4	0
Soybean	1 tsp	44	5	1	1	3	0
Sunflower	1 tsp	40	5	1	1	3	0
Vegetable	1 tsp	40	5	1	1	3	0
Pumpkin seeds, roasted	1 Tbsp	70	6	1	2	3	0
Salad dressing, regular (high sodium)	1 Tbsp	64	6	—	—	—	—
Salad dressing, light, reduced fat	2 Tbsp	80	6	1	—	—	—

	Serving	Cal.	Total fat (g)	Sat. fat (g)	Mono. fat (g)	Poly. fat (g)	Chol. (mg)
Sunflower seeds, dry roasted	1 Tbsp	47	4	0	1	3	0
Tartar sauce	2 tsp	46	5	1	1	3	4
Walnuts, halves	4	51	5	1	—	—	0

Fats, saturated

	Serving	Cal.	Total fat (g)	Sat. fat (g)	Mono. fat (g)	Poly. fat (g)	Chol. (mg)
Bacon, fried, drained	1 slice	35	3	1	1	0	5
Bacon grease	1 tsp	36	4	2	2	0	4
Butter, stick	1 tsp	36	4	3	1	0	11
Butter, whipped	2 tsp	40	5	3	—	—	13
Butter, reduced fat	1 Tbsp	50	6	4	—	—	20
Chitterlings, boiled	2 Tbsp	42	4	1	1	1	20
Coconut, shredded, dried, sweetened	2 Tbsp	52	4	3	0	0	0
Coconut, shredded, raw	2 Tbsp	35	3	3	0	0	0
Cream, half and half	1 Tbsp	39	4	2	1	0	11
Cream cheese, regular	1 Tbsp	49	5	3	1	0	15
Cream cheese, reduced fat	2 Tbsp	60	5	3	1	0	15
Lard	1 tsp	36	4	2	2	0	4
Salt pork, raw, cured	1/4 oz	52	6	2	3	1	6
Shortening	1 tsp	35	4	1	2	1	0
Sour cream, regular	2 Tbsp	52	5	3	2	0	10
Sour cream, reduced fat	3 Tbsp	45	4	3	1	0	15

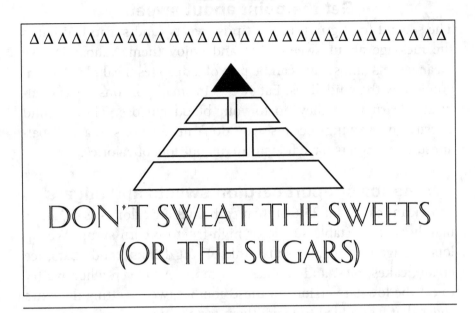

CHAPTER 9

DON'T SWEAT THE SWEETS (OR THE SUGARS)

What you will learn

▲ The new diabetes nutrition recommendations for sugars.

▲ Many names for "sugar."

▲ How sugars differ from sweets.

▲ How to be sugars wise.

▲ Ways to keep a lid on sweets while you satisfy your sweet tooth.

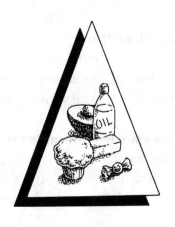

Get the point about sweets

The second food group in the tip is sweets (and sugars). What is the message about sweets? Eat and enjoy them. Whoa! Do we mean sweets and sugars can be part of a diabetes meal plan? Yes, if you follow the guidelines. Eat sweets in small portions occasionally and learn what they do to your blood glucose. The pyramid doesn't give servings because you don't need sweets in a well-balanced diet. Sweets have few nutrients but lots of calories.

America's report card on sweets and sugars

Americans eat about 25% of their carbohydrate calories as sugars—mainly sucrose (table sugar) or high-fructose corn syrup. We sip lots of sugars in regular soft drinks. Fruit drinks, candy bars, ice cream, cakes, pies, and cookies add more. And even when we try to eat the low-fat versions of these goodies, we're getting the extra sugar that was added to make them taste better.

What are sugars?

The term *sugars* does not refer just to the white granulated stuff. Think about the sugars you stock in your cupboard—white granulated sugar, brown sugar, maple syrup, molasses, and honey. Check out the sugars on food labels—high-fructose corn syrup, corn sweeteners, fruit juice concentrate, dextrose, and others. These are all sugars with 4 calories per gram—the same as other carbohydrates.

Natural and added sugars

We divide sugars into two categories—natural and added. Natural sugars are naturally a part of foods—sucrose in fruit or lactose in milk. Besides calories, these sugars give you carbohydrate, vitamins, and minerals.

Added sugars are sugars that are added to foods, such as high-fructose corn syrup in regular soda or fruit drinks. These sugars give you calories but few other nutrients. Knowing which sugars are which helps you make decisions in the supermarket.

Sugars and sweets—what's the difference?

Sweets contain sugars. However, sweets—cake, cookies, and pie—also have fats. It's the fat in sweets that makes the calorie count go sky high, not the sugars. If you need to lose weight or if you have problems with blood fats, sweets can cause you problems. The following list of desserts gives you an idea of how the calories add up when the fats are added:

Fat makes the difference in desserts

Food	Serving	Calories	Carbo-hydrate (g)	Fat (g)
Strawberry gelatin (regular)	1/2 cup	70	15	0
Strawberry pie (2 crust)	1 serving	360	49	18
Chocolate chips	1 Tbsp	66	9	4
Chocolate chip* cookies	2 small	248	28	14
Jelly beans	10/oz	66	26	0
Lemon meringue pie*	1 piece	362	49	16
Sugar, granulated	1 Tbsp	48	12	0
Ice cream* (regular, store brand)	1/2 cup	132	16	7

*Insignificant amount of saturated fat and cholesterol

Sugars and diabetes

Research studies show that, gram for gram, sugars, like table sugar, do not raise blood glucose any more quickly than do other carbohydrates, like potatoes, rice, or pasta. This research holds true for people with both types of diabetes.

A variety of factors influence how fast food is digested, such as a meal with a large amount of fat or fiber, lots of raw foods that take more time to digest, and eating slowly. Obviously, the blood glucose level at the time you eat and how much diabetes medication is in your body has a major impact, too.

Are fructose and honey better?

No. Fructose, honey, and fruit juice concentrates raise blood glucose just like white sugar does. The nutrition recommendations say that one is no better than another. They have about the same number of calories and, other than fructose, raise blood glucose at about the same speed. Fructose does raise blood glucose more slowly, but it might raise blood cholesterol, which is not good.

So now what?

The nutrition recommendations give first priority to the total amount of carbohydrate you eat, not where the carbohydrate comes from. The bottom line is carbohydrate is carbohydrate. Try to eat the same amount of carbohydrate at the same meals and snacks each day. For example, 45 g of carbohydrate at breakfast, and 60 g of carbohydrate at both lunch and dinner. Please be aware that you do not have to eat the same *foods* every day. Just count how many grams of carbohydrate—whether they come from beans, potatoes, or brownies. If you eat different *amounts* of carbohydrate each day, it will be difficult for you to control your blood glucose levels.

When you choose to eat a sweet, you need to substitute it for other carbohydrates in your meal plan. To decide how many sugars and sweets to eat, you'll need to answer these questions:

▲ Is my blood glucose out of control and glycated hemoglobin higher than desirable?
▲ Do I need to lose weight, so I cannot afford a lot of calories as sugars and sweets?
▲ Are my blood fats—total cholesterol, LDL, HDL, and triglycerides—out of control?
▲ How much do I enjoy sugars and sweets, and how often do I want a small serving?

▲ Can I be more physically active after eating sugars and sweets to burn the extra calories?

Get sugars wise

▲ Prioritize your personal diabetes goals. Which comes first: blood glucose control, weight loss, or lower blood fats? Your priorities dictate how you strike the balance with sugars and sweets.

▲ Choose a few favorite desserts and decide how often to eat them in the light of your personal diabetes goals—maybe twice a week, just when dining out, or only at a special celebration.

▲ Note the calories, total fat, saturated fat, and cholesterol of the desserts you prefer. Then make your choices with these numbers and your diabetes goals in mind.

▲ Satisfy your sweet tooth with a small portion of your favorite sweet.

▲ Split a dessert in a restaurant.

▲ Take advantage of smaller portions when you can.

▲ Use Nutrition Facts on the food label to get the grams of carbohydrate per serving. You need this information to swap a sweet food with another carbohydrate in your meal plan.

▲ Check the Nutrition Facts for the grams of sugars under total carbohydrate, and read the ingredient list to find natural and added sugars.

▲ When you eat a sweet, test your blood glucose to see its affect. You might find that, due to the fat content, the same quantity of ice cream raises your blood glucose more slowly than frozen yogurt, which contains less fat and more carbohydrate. Let this information help you decide what sweets to eat and when.

▲ Keep an eye on glycated hemoglobin and blood lipid levels to see whether eating more sweets leads to a rise in the numbers.

How many servings

You do not need to eat sugars to get nutrients. You automatically eat some sugars because sugars are in many foods—from raisins and milk to ketchup, bread, and salad dressing. The recommendation is to eat sweets in moderation. Look at this sample 1-day meal plan to see how sweets are included. In all there are 75 grams of sugars (16% of the calories). Remember that includes the natural sugars from fruits, milk, and yogurt as well as the added sugars in the frozen yogurt. There is one serving in bold type. Nutrient information is on page 18.

Breakfast
1 whole oat bran English muffin
1/2 large grapefruit
2 Tbsp light cream cheese

Lunch
1 pita pocket, 6" across, cut in half to fill
1/3 medium sliced tomato
1/3 cup sliced cucumbers
1/2 cup sliced large carrots or whole baby carrots
1 oz lean ham or turkey
1 oz part-skim Swiss cheese
Mustard to spread on bread
1 cup of low-fat/skim milk

Afternoon Snack
1 cup nonfat fruited yogurt sweetened with low-calorie sweetener
2 small tangerines

Dinner
5 oz dry red wine
1 cup spaghetti
1 whole wheat dinner roll
1 cup tomato sauce made with
    3/4 cup prepared tomato sauce
    1/3 cup onions
    1/3 cup peppers
    2 tsp canola oil (use to sauté onions and peppers)
    2 oz ground turkey, browned and drained (3 oz raw)

Spinach salad with
  1 cup spinach
  1/3 cup sliced mushrooms
  1 tsp purple onion
  2 Tbsp reduced-fat French salad dressing

Evening Snack
  1/2 cup light ice cream (1 serving)
  1 1/4 cups whole strawberries, sliced

A serving of sugars and sweets

The chart at the end of the chapter shows the serving size for sweets with information on calories, carbohydrate, total fat, saturated fat, and cholesterol content. You can see that the calories and fat from sweets add up quickly.

Get to know yourself

If you want to make your eating habits healthier, you need to learn what you're eating now. Ask yourself these questions:
▲ How many times a day or a week do I eat sweets?
▲ What foods do I eat that contain sugars?
▲ How often and in what quantity do I eat these foods?
▲ What are my favorite sweets?
▲ How often would I like to eat sweets?

Change...one step at a time

Use your answers to the questions above to set some goals for blood glucose control, weight, and blood lipids. If you've been staying away from sweets, you can pick one, find the nutrition information, and substitute it for an equal amount of carbohydrate in your meal plan. (This is one reason you need a meal plan and to count the grams of carbohydrate that you eat each day.)

If you eat too many sweets and are battling the bulge, you might want to make a contract with yourself about what sweets you will eat, how often, and in what quantity. If having sweets in the house is too difficult, then eat sweets only in restaurants or in ice cream or frozen yogurt shops.

Easy ways to keep a lid on sugars and sweets

▲ Use no-sugar or low-sugar jelly or jams or small amounts of regular jelly or jam.

▲ Use low-calorie sweeteners in hot or cold beverages or on cereal or fruit.

▲ Buy sweets in small quantities.

▲ Do not buy or order sweets that you will have difficulty eating in small quantities.

▲ Try half of your usual portion.

▲ Leave out some of the sugar in recipes.

▲ Take advantage of low-calorie, no-sugar foods: diet gelatin, powdered drink mix, and no-sugar jelly.

▲ Watch out for beverages with lots of sugar—fruit drinks, fruit-flavored drinks, sweetened seltzers, and sweetened iced tea.

Now you know

▲ The difference between sugars and sweets.

▲ The new recommendations about sugars and sweets for people with diabetes.

▲ How to decide how much sugars or sweets to eat.

▲ Tactics to satisfy your sweet tooth.

Scenario

Meet John. He is an active high school senior who has had type I diabetes for 4 years. He plays several high school sports and is in the middle of basketball season on the varsity team. He takes insulin four times a day, before each meal and at bedtime. He finds it easier to adjust food and medication with the flexibility of taking a shot of regular insulin at meals.

John is 6'2" and weighs 192 pounds, so he needs at least 3000 calories a day. He actually has to work to keep his weight up. Since the new guidelines about sweets came out, John met with his dietitian. He would like to have some. His dietitian says he can because he requires so many calories daily, knows how to adjust his regular insulin based on the amount of carbohydrate he eats, has normal blood lipid levels, and has his diabetes under good control.

John listed peach cobbler, butter pecan ice cream, and chocolate chip cookies as his favorite sweets. She showed him how to substitute a sweet into his meal plan by eating 1 to 2 fewer starches and less fat in the meal to keep the impact on blood glucose about the same.

They decided he can eat a sweet at dinner on the days that he has a basketball practice or game in the afternoon. Other times, a sweet might fit in lunch or as a snack before a practice. They decide that three or four times a week is his limit.

To see how sweets affect his diabetes control, he will test his blood glucose about 1 1/2 hours after eating sweets and have his glycated hemoglobin checked quarterly, as he does now. He will also keep an eye on his blood lipid levels to catch any changes.

Scenario

Meet Sharon. She is a 67-year-old retired school teacher. Sharon was recently diagnosed with type II diabetes. She has about 25 pounds to lose, but her first goal is to lose 10 pounds. Besides high blood glucose (glycated hemoglobin 8.7%), she also has high LDL (bad cholesterol) and high triglycerides.

Sharon has a sweet tooth; she is used to having a "sweet treat" every day. Since she met with an RD she is trying to eat 1200–1400 calories a day, with no more than 35–45 g of fat (about 30%).

Sharon and her dietitian have fit in a sweet treat once or twice a week. She only eats them when she is away from her home, because she believes she will eat too much if sweets are in her house. Her choices are often a small serving of frozen yogurt, light ice cream, or splitting dessert in a restaurant when she eats out. Her dietitian suggested she keep sugar-free hot cocoa mix, popsicles, and gingersnaps around to satisfy her sweet tooth.

	Serving	Calor.	Carbo-hydrate (g)	Total Fat (g)	Sat. fat (g)	Choles-terol (mg)
Sweets						
Angel food cake	1/12	142	32	0	0	0
Brownie, small	1	115	18	5	1	5
Cake, unfrosted, 2" square	1	97	17	3	1	18
Cake, frosted, 2" square	1	175	29	6	2	18
Candy bar, milk chocolate	1 1/2 oz	240	25	14	8	10
Cheesecake, plain, from recipe	3 oz	303	21	22	12	102
Chocolate syrup	2 Tbsp	110	25	1	0	0
Cookies, fat free	2	68	16	0	0	0
Cookie, 3" diameter	1	142	19	7	2	10
Cookies, small, 1 3/4" diameter	2	114	15	6	2	8
Cookie, sandwich with cream filling	2	94	14	4	1	1
Cupcake, frosted, small	1	172	28	6	2	1
Custard, made with 2% milk	1/2 cup	149	24	4	2	74
Donut, plain cake	1	198	23	11	2	18
Donut, glazed, 3 3/4" diameter	2 oz	242	27	14	4	4
Gelatin, regular (Jello)	1/2 cup	80	19	0	0	0
Gingersnaps	3	87	16	2	0	0
Honey	1 tsp	20	5	0	0	0
Ice cream, 10% fat	1/2 cup	133	16	7	5	29
Ice cream, light	1/2 cup	100	14	4	3	25

	Serving	Calor.	Carbo-hydrate (g)	Total Fat (g)	Sat. fat (g)	Choles-terol (mg)
Ice cream, no sugar added	1/2 cup	100	13	4	3	15
Ice cream, fat free	1/2 cup	90	20	0	0	0
Jam or preserves, regular	1 Tbsp	48	13	0	0	0
Jelly, regular	1 Tbsp	52	14	0	0	0
Marshmallows	2	50	12	0	0	0
Pie, fruit, 2 crusts	1/6	290	43	13	2	0
Pie, pumpkin or custard	1/8	168	19	8	1	21
Pound cake, frozen	1/10	70	17	6	3	66
Pudding, regular	1/2 cup	144	27	3	2	9
Pudding, sugar free, from low-fat milk	1/2 cup	90	13	2	2	9
Sherbet	1/2 cup	132	29	2	1	5
Sugar, white	1 tsp	16	4	0	0	0
Sugar, brown, packed	1 tsp	17	5	0	0	0
Sweet roll or Danish, 2 1/2 oz	1	293	38	9	3	0
Syrup, maple, regular	1 Tbsp	52	13	0	0	0
Syrup, pancake, light	2 Tbsp	50	13	0	0	0
Syrup, pancake, regular	1 Tbsp	57	15	0	0	0
Toaster pastry, low fat, all flavors	1	171	40	0	0	0
Yogurt, frozen, low fat	1/3 cup	66	14	1	1	3
Yogurt frozen, fat free	1/3 cup	60	12	0	0	0
Vanilla wafers	5	88	15	3	1	12

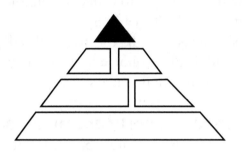

CHAPTER 10

ALCOHOL AT THE TIP-SY

What you will learn

▲ Health and safety concerns.

▲ Special health and safety concerns with diabetes.

▲ The when and how to drink alcohol if you take medications that lower blood glucose.

▲ How much alcohol to drink if weight loss is your goal.

▲ The calories in alcoholic beverages.

▲ Tips to sip by.

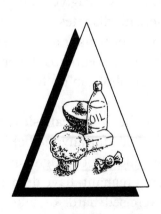

The last of the three...alcohol

The third resident of the tip is alcohol. What is the message about alcohol for you? If you choose to drink alcohol, limit the amount, and drink it with a meal. The carbohydrates in the meal will help keep your blood glucose up. In the pages ahead you'll find out whether you should drink alcohol, and if so, when. For individual advice, ask your health-care providers.

America's report card on alcohol

Americans continue to drink quite a bit. Interestingly, the kind of alcohol we drink has changed—more wine and beer and less hard liquor. And now we have designated drivers for an evening.

No need for alcohol

Alcohol offers no essential nutrients. Even though alcohol is not nutritionally necessary, you can have some if it mixes with your diabetes goals and you practice safety measures.

The downside

Too many people drink too much. This causes many problems, from cancer to traffic accidents. From both a health and safety standpoint, the message is "less is best and none is better."

Alcohol has 7 calories per gram and few nutrients. Too much alcohol can pack on the pounds. Alcohol can also wreak havoc on blood lipid levels and make triglycerides rise. These are often already high in people with diabetes, especially those with type II. However, a small amount of regular alcohol can raise good cholesterol (HDL) to a slight degree. Perhaps the best-known health hazard is the damage that alcohol can do to the liver. This can lead to cirrhosis and death.

Alcohol's effect on the brain can slow physical and mental reactions. This is dangerous for anyone behind the wheel of a car, where quick reactions and good judgment are vital. You should avoid alcohol if you are pregnant, have diabetic neuropathy (nerve disease), have just exercised hard, or take prescription or over-the-counter medications that should not be mixed with alcohol.

Diabetes and alcohol

If you have diabetes and are on diabetes medications that lower blood glucose, be warned. One of the things alcohol does is keep the liver from making glucose. So, if you drink at the same time insulin or a diabetes pill is lowering blood glucose, you could get into trouble. Don't drink when your blood glucose is low, your insulin or diabetes pill is working hardest, or your stomach is empty. Alcohol not only causes low blood glucose (hypoglycemia) shortly after drinking, it can continue to cause it for 8–12 hours. Test your blood glucose and eat your planned meal to prevent low blood glucose.

The symptoms of too much alcohol and of hypoglycemia are similar. You don't want people to confuse these two, because they might not give the proper treatment when you need it.

Less often, alcohol can cause blood glucose to rise. This is due to the calories from carbohydrates in some alcoholic beverages such as beer and wine or the calories from a mixer such as orange juice. So, if you have a drink with a meal and your diabetes medication is not peaking, alcohol might make your blood glucose rise.

For people with diabetes who must balance medication, blood glucose testing, and food, alcohol may lead to poor decisions about your diabetes care. Plus, it can weaken your desire to eat healthfully.

How much is too much?

How much alcohol can you drink and when? According to the diabetes nutrition guidelines, if your diabetes is under control, you may drink a moderate amount of alcohol. A moderate amount is 1 drink each day. One drink equals a 12-oz beer, 5 oz of wine, or 1 1/2 oz of whiskey. People on insulin or people on diabetes medications who are not overweight can drink this amount of alcohol in addition to their meal plan. If you are not on insulin and particularly if you are overweight, you can substitute alcohol into your meal plan as a fat. Ask your dietitian for help with this.

How many servings

Make your decision based on your answers to these questions:

▲ Have I ever abused alcohol or do I believe I could?

▲ Is my blood glucose under control?

▲ Do I take diabetes medication? If yes, how often do I experience low blood glucose, and do I know how to treat it?

▲ Have I had problems with alcohol causing me to have low blood glucose reactions? If yes, when, what kind, and how much alcohol did I drink? How did I treat the hypoglycemia?

▲ Do I need to lose some weight and therefore need to count calories?

▲ Is my blood triglyceride level high?

▲ Do I enjoy an alcoholic beverage, and how often do I want a small amount?

▲ Do I have a physically active lifestyle to help burn the extra calories?

This sample 1-day food plan shows how you can include a small amount of alcohol in your meal plan. Note, the glass of wine is part of the meal to prevent low blood glucose. This amount of alcohol is about 100 calories (5% of the day's calories). Nutrient information is on page 18.

Breakfast
> 1 whole oat bran English muffin
> 1/2 large grapefruit
> 2 Tbsp light cream cheese

Lunch
> 1 pita pocket, 6" across, cut in half to fill
> 1/3 medium sliced tomato
> 1/3 cup sliced cucumbers
> 1/2 cup sliced large carrots or whole baby carrots
> 1 oz lean ham or turkey
> 1 oz part-skim Swiss cheese
> Mustard to spread on bread
> 1 cup of low-fat/skim milk

Afternoon Snack
1 cup nonfat fruited yogurt sweetened with low-calorie sweetener

2 small tangerines

Dinner
5 oz dry red wine (1 serving)

1 cup spaghetti

1 whole wheat dinner roll

1 cup tomato sauce made with

    3/4 cup prepared tomato sauce

    1/3 cup onions

    1/3 cup peppers

    2 tsp canola oil (use to sauté onions and peppers)

    2 oz ground turkey, browned and drained (3 oz raw)

Spinach salad with

    1 cup spinach

    1/3 cup sliced mushrooms

    1 tsp purple onion

    2 Tbsp reduced-fat French salad dressing

Evening Snack
1/2 cup light ice cream

1 1/4 cups whole strawberries, sliced

A serving of alcohol

A serving of alcohol is one 12-oz beer, or 5 oz of wine, or 1 1/2 oz of distilled spirits, such as gin or whiskey. Alcohol has 7 calories in each gram. This is close to the 9 calories per gram of fat. The calories from alcohol can add up quickly.

Calories not equal

A serving of light beer, wine, gin, or whiskey has about 100 calories. The calories climb when you opt for a regular beer over light beer or a premixed wine cooler instead of a glass of wine. Nonalcoholic beer and wine are not light in calories either. Check the label or ask your dietitian for help with your choices.

You add more calories when you add mixers. To keep a low score on the calories and sugars from mixers stick with these: club soda, mineral water, diet tonic water, water, diet soda, tomato or V8 juice, Bloody Mary mix, or coffee (for a hot drink).

Alcohol adds flavor, not fat

A bit of wine, sherry, or liqueur can enhance the taste of foods and not add fat and calories. Alcohol is a wonderful low-fat cooking ingredient. You might stock red and white cooking wine, sherry, and liqueurs (clear ones, not creamy) in your pantry.

Here are a few ideas: add sherry to a marinade for chicken or meat, pour red cooking wine in a tomato sauce, use white cooking wine in a poaching liquid, add orange liqueur to a fruit salad, dress up coffee with a spot of hazelnut liqueur, or drizzle a tablespoon of raspberry liqueur on frozen yogurt.

Get to know yourself

To change your eating habits, you need to know what they are. Ask yourself these questions about alcohol:

▲ How many times a day or a week do I drink alcohol?

▲ What types of alcohol do I drink?

▲ Do I mix alcohol with a mixer, such as juice, soda, or tonic water?

▲ How often would I like to drink alcohol?

▲ How many drinks are reasonable when I drink?

Change...one step at a time

Use your answers to the questions above to set your goals. Your goals for drinking alcohol will depend on your blood glucose control, weight, and blood lipids. Maybe you choose to limit where you drink alcohol. You decide to drink only when you eat an evening meal in restaurants and not at home.

Tips to sip by

▲ Drink only when blood glucose is under control.

▲ Test blood glucose to help you decide whether you should

drink and when you need to eat something.

▲ Wear or carry identification stating that you have diabetes.

▲ Sip a drink slowly to make it last.

▲ Have a no-calorie beverage on the side to quench your thirst.

▲ If you take diabetes medications that can cause low blood glucose, always have a snack or meal with the alcohol.

▲ If you do not take diabetes medications and have some pounds to shed, substitute alcohol for fats in your meal plan.

▲ Ask an RD to help you fit alcohol into your food plan.

▲ Do not drive for several hours after you drink alcohol.

Now you know

▲ When it is and is not safe to drink alcohol with diabetes.

▲ The calories and nutrients in alcohol.

▲ How much alcohol to drink and how to fit it in your meal plan.

▲ How alcohol can enhance the flavor of food without adding fat.

Scenario

Meet John. He has had type II diabetes for 3 years and is now 47 years old. He has worked out a 2000-calorie meal plan with his dietitian and takes a diabetes pill (that can cause hypoglycemia) twice a day. He tries to fit in a 1-mile walk two times a week.

With this plan, over the last 15 months, he shed 12 pounds, and his blood glucose control has improved. His glycated hemoglobin decreased from a high of 8.6% to 7.3%. Now he needs to lower his triglycerides. He has about 16 more pounds to lose before he reaches what he calls his "fighting weight."

John travels a lot for work and finds himself at business dinners 3 nights a week. He usually has a cocktail and wine and, on occasion, an after-dinner liqueur. On the weekend, he might drink a few beers or several glasses of wine at a restaurant or while watching TV. See how fast the calories add up from one of John's business dinners:

Cocktail: 1 rum and diet cola (1 1/2 oz rum)—96 calories

Wine: 1 glass dry white wine (5 oz)—98 calories

After-dinner liqueur: Kahlua (1 1/2 oz)—175 calories

Almost 400 calories just from alcohol. That's about 20% of John's 2000 calories for the day—more than he should allot to alcohol.

John recognizes that the alcohol is not helping him lose weight or lower his triglycerides. And he had an early-morning low blood glucose level (after a business dinner). He knows it's time to start lowering the amount of alcohol he drinks.

He'll drink only light beer and stop at 2 beers a day. When he is on business trips, he'll drink either a cocktail or a glass of wine with dinner and skip the after-dinner liqueur. When he is out to dinner on the weekend, he will split half a bottle of wine or order a glass of wine.

He will make sure to have a 0-calorie drink on the side, and he will check his blood glucose before bed after drinking in the evening. He will eat an additional snack if his blood glucose is below 90 mg/dl.

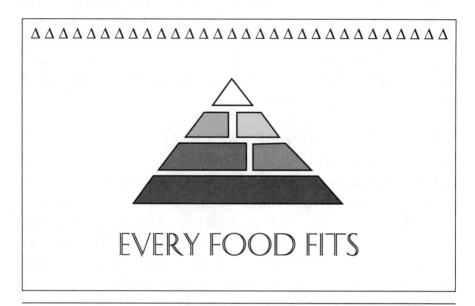

CHAPTER 11

EVERY FOOD FITS

What you will learn

▲ The meaning of mixed or combination foods.

▲ How to fit your favorite mixed or combination foods into the food pyramid.

▲ How to design healthy and balanced meals with convenience foods.

▲ The meaning of free foods.

▲ Reasonable portions of free foods.

Where, oh where

You have read a lot in the preceding chapters about foods that fit nicely into the different food groups. It makes perfect sense— apples in the fruit group; barley in the grains, beans, and starchy vegetable group; or pork chops in the meat group. For lunch, have 2 starches (2 slices of whole-grain bread), 1 fruit (2 small tangerines), and so forth.

But where do foods like bean burritos, beef stew, or Chinese chicken with vegetables fit? Bean burritos, for example, have ingredients from several food groups—beans and tortillas from the grains, beans, and starchy vegetables; cheese from the meat and others; lettuce, onion, and tomato from the vegetables; and salsa from the free foods. Macaroni and cheese has mainly starches and, depending on the recipe, milk or fats. Ask your dietitian for help figuring the pyramid servings in some of your favorite recipes. With practice, you'll be able to fit combination dishes into pyramid servings even in a restaurant.

With a diabetes cookbook

Cookbooks written for people with diabetes have nutrition information and diabetes exchanges. The combination foods are figured out for you. In the future, you may find that some cookbooks provide the servings according to the food pyramid. In most cases, you can use exchanges to figure food pyramid servings. It's easy. You can make a one to one swap between exchanges and servings from the food pyramid, except for meats. One meat exchange serving is 1 oz and 1 pyramid serving is 2–3 oz of meat.

With a food label in hand

It is also easy to fit convenience or prepared foods into your meal plan. Perhaps you want to eat a can of pasta with tomato sauce or a frozen entree like chicken teriyaki with vegetables over rice. From the Nutrition Facts, you know the grams of carbohydrate, protein, and fat per serving, and from the ingredients list, you know which ingredients contribute these nutrients. Use the two lists to figure out the servings from the food pyramid.

You can figure out the number of pyramid servings in a dish. Just subtract the grams of carbohydrate, protein, and fat in one pyramid serving from the grams of each on the food label. Use the following example of a frozen entree of stuffed cabbage and carrots over rice to practice. The Nutrition Facts tell you that there are

> 38 g of carbohydrate,
> 23 g of protein, and
> 6 g of fat

in one serving of cabbage, carrots, and rice.

You know (from chapter 4) that 1 pyramid serving of starch has 15 g of carbohydrate and 3 g of protein. Subtract these amounts from the amounts on the food label to see whether you have 1 pyramid serving of starch. You do, and you have 23 g of carbohydrate left over. That means you have another starch serving.

	Carbohydrate	Protein	Fat
1 serving on the food label	38 g	23 g	6 g
1 pyramid starch serving	−15 g	−3 g	0 g
	23 g	20 g	6 g
Another starch serving	−15 g	−3 g	0 g
	8 g	17 g	6 g

Now you have 8 g of carbohydrate and 17 g of protein left. The amount of protein tells you to check for a serving of meat and others. One pyramid lean-meat serving has 0 g carbohydrate, 14 g of protein, and 6 g of fat. Subtract these amounts from your food-label amounts.

	Carbohydrate	Protein	Fat
Left in the rice dish	8 g	17 g	6 g
1 pyramid serving meat	−0 g	−14 g	6 g
	8 g	3 g	0 g

You have 8 g of carbohydrate left over and very little protein. Now check for 1 pyramid serving of vegetables (5 g carbohydrate, 2 g protein) by subtracting these amounts of carbohydrate and protein from the food-label amounts you have left over.

	Carbohydrate	Protein	Fat
	8 g	3 g	
1 pyramid serving vegetables	−5 g	−2 g	
	3 g	1 g	

The rice dish has 3 pyramid food groups in it: 2 starch servings, 1 meat serving, and 1 vegetable serving. With this information, you can fit it into your meal plan. To balance this meal, add slices of cucumber and tomatoes or a green salad and a piece of fruit. You'll learn more about using Nutrition Facts in Part 2.

When you dine out

It is more of a challenge to figure out what is in restaurant dishes. It helps if you have a detailed description on the menu rather than just the name. If there is no description, ask about the ingredients, the way they're prepared, and the serving size before you order. Ask as many questions as you need to help you determine what to order and how to fit a serving into your meal plan. Don't forget to ask for a doggie bag if the quantity of food is more than you need.

The more practice you get fitting recipes and convenience foods into your meal plan, the easier it will be to fit restaurant foods. Here is an example from a Mexican restaurant:

Black bean soup, 1 cup	2 starches
	small amount fat
Beef fajitas (split the meat and order extra tortillas)	
2 tortillas	2 starches
3 oz beef	1 meat, medium fat
1/2–3/4 cup sautéed onions and peppers in oil	1–2 vegetables with 5 g fat
2 Tbsp guacamole	5 g fat
1/2–3/4 cup lettuce, tomato, and fresh onion	1 vegetable
4 Tbsp salsa	free food

A serving of mixed foods

The chart at the end of the chapter shows the servings for a variety of combination foods with their calorie, carbohydrate, protein, fat, saturated fat, and sodium content.

Convenience foods—healthy you say?

Convenience foods are not as healthy as the same item made at home. Generally, they are higher in sodium and have many more additives and preservatives. Does that mean you should not eat them? No. Would it be better to make all of your meals from fresh fruits, vegetables, grains, and meats? Yes. But most people can't do that. So, a few convenience foods can be part of a healthy meal plan. You'll probably do better to fit some convenience foods into your meal plan instead of a fast-food or restaurant meal.

Design meals with convenience foods

Many convenience foods are combination dishes and you can make them part of your meal plan. (See page 131.) The Nutrition Facts help you figure out the number of pyramid servings in the food. The stuffed cabbage over rice in the example on page 124 has 2 starch servings, 1 meat serving, and 1 vegetable serving. Here are a few more examples:

Breakfast with frozen waffle for a meal plan with

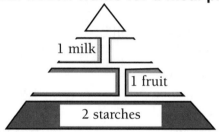

2 frozen waffles	2 starches, 8 g fat
1 1/4 cups sliced strawberries	1 fruit
2 Tbsp of light maple syrup	sweet
1 cup skim milk	1 milk

Lunch with frozen cheese and tomato pizza for meal plan with

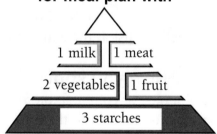

2 slices pizza topped with red peppers, tomatoes, and mushrooms	3 starches, 1 meat, 2 vegetables
1 cup fat-free, sugar-free strawberry yogurt	1 milk
1 small banana sliced into yogurt	1 fruit

Dinner with frozen entree for meal plan with

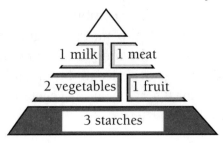

Chicken Oriental Stir-Fry — 2 starches, 1 vegetable, 1 meat

1 small whole-wheat dinner roll or
   1 slice whole-grain bread — 1 starch

Salad with lettuce, cucumbers,
   carrots, and sliced tomato — 1 vegetable

1 tsp extra-virgin olive oil — 5 g fat

2 Tbsp balsamic vinegar — free food

1 cup skim milk — 1 milk

What about free foods?

The last group of foods on your meal plan are the so-called free foods. Free foods do not have a space on the food pyramid because they have too few calories per serving to count. One serving of a free food has less than 20 calories or less than 5 g of carbohydrate. Spread free foods out over the meals for the day to keep them from having an effect on your blood glucose. Don't eat too much, even if they are "free." Check the list at the end of this chapter.

Now you know

▲ The definition of mixed or combination foods.

▲ How to fit combination foods into the food pyramid.

▲ About free foods.

Scenario

Meet Ray. Ray is 72 years old and has been a widower about a year. He has had type II diabetes for 3 years and takes diabetes pills before breakfast and dinner. Ray's wife did all the cooking, so he stocks a few frozen meals and bags of frozen vegetables in the freezer and keeps some canned goods on the shelf. Otherwise, he eats at nearby cafeterias.

Recently, Ray met with an RD he saw after he was first diagnosed with diabetes. His doctor asked him to go because he has gained 8 pounds since his wife died and his blood glucose is climbing. The RD pointed out that Ray chooses some high-fat foods. For convenience foods, Ray buys the regular type of frozen meals and chooses chicken pot pie, meat loaf with gravy and potatoes, and lasagna. For vegetables, he chooses spinach souffle, peas and onions in butter sauce, and broccoli in cheese sauce.

The RD suggested that Ray purchase products that are lower in fat and calories and have smaller portions. She said it is better to buy vegetables without cream, cheese, or butter sauce. If Ray wants to put a bit of butter or margarine on the vegetables after they are cooked, that is fine. A squeeze of lemon or lime is even better.

In the cafeteria Ray should order an entree, starch, 2 vegetables, and a salad. Some of the entrees that Ray could order are meatloaf with gravy, roast beef, roasted chicken, and fried fish. The RD suggested that Ray ask for a take-home container when he orders his meal. When he first sits down, he can put half the entree in the container to save for another meal. Then he can enjoy a reasonable amount of meat, starches, and vegetables. She encouraged him to watch out for the fats in fried foods, butter, sour cream, and creamy sauces on vegetables.

They discussed how many servings from the food pyramid Ray should eat each day and how some of his food selections fit in. She emphasized that 2–3 oz of meat is 1 serving and Ray's cafeteria choices are closer to 6–8 oz of meat—perfect to split into two portions.

Scenario

Meet Sandy. She is 25 years old, is single, and has had type I diabetes for 8 years. She recently started her first job after finishing law school. She is adjusting to her new life as a hard-working attorney in a busy office.

Sandy tries to stay on track with her diabetes. She eats a quick bowl of cereal with fruit or pops an English muffin into the toaster and grabs a banana to eat on the way. She takes lunch from home—a sandwich, piece of fruit, and a handful of pretzels. The days she goes out with colleagues or clients, she ends up overeating.

By the time she gets home at night, she is too tired and hungry to spend time cooking. She finds that the healthier convenience meals are satisfying and quick. She learned how to fit these meals into her meal plan in a class she attended recently. In general, they are 1 serving of meat, 1 starch, and 1 vegetable.

Her meal plan for dinner calls for 1 serving of meat, 2 starches, 2–3 vegetables, 1 fruit, and 1 milk. Sandy knows that along with the frozen entree she needs a whole wheat roll or crackers for another starch and a salad, sliced tomato, or handful of baby carrots for another vegetable. She adds a cup of skim milk and has a piece of fruit soon after dinner. Other evenings, Sandy grabs a quick meal out with friends or gets a takeout meal at a pizza shop or rotisserie-chicken shop.

	Serv.	Cal.	Carbo-hydrate (g)	Prot. (g)	Total fat (g)	Sat. fat (g)	Sod-ium (mg)
Main Courses							
Chili con carne	1 cup	256	22	25	8	3	1007
Chow mein, beef	2 cups	160	13	16	3	1	2373
Lasagna	8 oz	302	27	22	12	7	885
Macaroni and cheese	1 cup	228	26	9	4	4	730
Pizza, cheese, thin crust, 10"	1/4	317	28	14	17	7	770
Pizza, meat topping, thin crust, 10"	1/4	368	29	15	21	7	1000
Pot pie, individual, double crust	1	450	35	13	28	7	778
Spaghetti, tomato sauce, meatballs	1 cup	258	29	12	10	2	1220
Tuna noodle casserole	9 oz	259	34	13	8	3	1043
Salisbury steak, gravy, mashed potatoes	11 oz	500	26	23	34	7	600
Turkey, gravy, mashed. potatoes, dressing, vegetables	11 oz	390	35	18	20	3	1110
Soups							
Bean	1 cup	116	20	6	2	0	1198
Beef noodle	1 cup	83	9	5	3	1	952
Chicken noodle	1 cup	75	9	4	3	1	1106
Cream of celery, made with water	1 cup	90	9	2	6	1	949
Cream of mushroom, made with water	1 cup	129	9	2	9	2	1032
Split pea	1 cup	95	14	5	2	1	504
Tomato, made with water	1 cup	85	17	2	2	0	871
Vegetable beef	1 cup	78	10	6	2	1	956

	Serving	Cal.	Carbo-hydrate (g)	Sodium (mg)
Free foods: low fat or fat free				
Cream cheese, fat free	1 Tbsp	15	1	80
Creamer, nondairy, liquid	1 Tbsp	18	2	5
Creamer, nondairy, powder	1 tsp	22	2	7
Mayonnaise, fat free	1 Tbsp	10	2	105
Mayonnaise, low fat, light	1 Tbsp	40	3	120
Margarine, fat free	4 Tbsp	20	0	360
Margarine, low fat, light	1 Tbsp	50	0	60
Miracle Whip, nonfat	1 Tbsp	15	3	105
Miracle Whip, light, reduced calorie	1 Tbsp	45	2	95
No-stick cooking spray	1 spray	2	0	0
Salad dressing, fat free (check sodium)	1 Tbsp	20	5	145
Salad dressing, Italian, fat free (check sodium)	2 Tbsp	12	3	420
Salsa	1/4 cup	14	3	168
Sour cream, light	1 Tbsp	18	2	15
Sour cream, fat free	1 Tbsp	15	3	20
Whipped topping	2 Tbsp	24	2	2
Whipped topping, light	2 Tbsp	19	2	2
Free foods: low sugar or sugar free				
Candy, hard, sugar free	1 piece	20	5	0
Fruit spread, 100% fruit	1 Tbsp	43	11	5
Gelatin dessert, sugar free	1/2 cup	8	1	56
Gelatin, unflavored	1 tsp	23	0	14
Jam or jelly, low sugar	2 tsp	15	4	4
Sugar substitutes (with saccharin or aspartame)	1 pkt	4	1	2
Syrup, sugar free	2 Tbsp	18	5	53

	Serving	Cal.	Carbo-hydrate (g)	Sodium (mg)
Drinks				
Broth type	1 cup	28	1	779
Bouillon or broth, granular/ cubes (check sodium)	1 tsp	5	1	576
Bouillon or broth, low-sodium granules	1 tsp	13	2	5
Carbonated water	1 cup	0	0	3
Cocoa powder, unsweetened	1 Tbsp	11	3	0
Coffee, brewed	3/4 cup	4	1	4
Club soda	12 oz	0	0	75
Diet soft drinks, sugar free	12 oz	2	0	21
Drink mixes, sugar free	1 cup	7	2	0
Mineral water	1 cup	0	0	3
Tea, brewed	3/4 cup	2	0	5
Tonic water, sugar free	1 cup	0	0	35
Condiments				
Bacon bits	1 tsp	10	0	104
Bacon bits, imitation	1 tsp	13	1	45
Barbeque sauce	1 Tbsp	18	4	120
Catsup, tomato	1 Tbsp	16	4	178
Chutney	2 tsp	17	5	25
Horseradish	1 Tbsp	6	1	14
Lemon juice	1 Tbsp	3	1	3
Lime juice	1 Tbsp	4	1	0
Mustard, prepared	1 tsp	4	0	63
Pickle relish	1 Tbsp	14	3	90
Pickles, dill, large (check sodium)	1 1/2	18	4	1256
Seafood cocktail sauce	1 Tbsp	15	3	170
Soy sauce (check sodium)	1 Tbsp	7	1	1024

	Serving	Cal.	Carbo-hydrate (g)	Sodium (mg)
Soy sauce, light (check sodium)	1 Tbsp	7	1	605
Sweet and sour sauce	1 Tbsp	17	5	95
Taco sauce	1 Tbsp	7	2	102
Teriyaki sauce				
Vinegars				
Balsamic	1 Tbsp	10	3	0
Cider	1/4 cup	8	4	1
Red wine	1 Tbsp	6	1	1
Rice wine	1 Tbsp	20	5	240

Seasonings

	Serving	Cal.	Carbo-hydrate (g)	Sodium (mg)
Cilantro	1/4 cup	1	0	1
Garlic	1 clove	1	0	0
Herbs, fresh	1 Tbsp	15	4	5
Herbs, dried	1 tsp	5	1	0
Pimiento, canned, solids and liquid	1 Tbsp	3	1	0
Parsley, raw	2 Tbsp	3	1	5
Spices	1 Tbsp	5–10	1–2	0
Tabasco sauce	1 tsp	1	0	30
Wine, used in cooking	1/4 cup	40	2	340
Worcestershire sauce	1 tsp	4	1	49

△△△△△△△△△△△△△△△△△△△△△△△△△△△△△△△△△△△

PART TWO

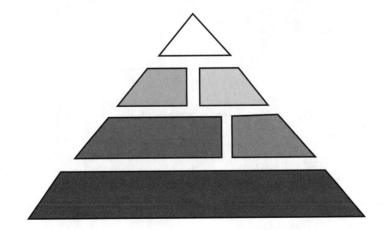

△△△△△△△△△△△△△△△△△△△△△△△△△△△△△△△△△△△

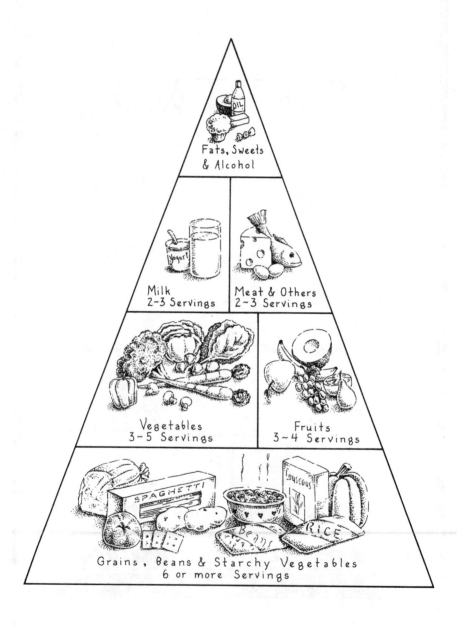

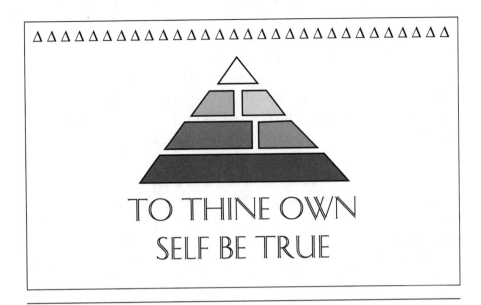

CHAPTER 12

TO THINE OWN
SELF BE TRUE

What you will learn

▲ Managing diabetes in our fast paced world is our day-to-day challenge.

▲ Being honest with yourself and your health-care providers is vitally important.

▲ The importance of keeping records and how to fit recordkeeping into your daily schedule.

▲ What realistic goals are and how to set them.

▲ Where to find help with using the Diabetes Food Pyramid.

Managing diabetes: a tough job

Recognize and acknowledge the time you take to manage your diabetes. Pat yourself on the back. Listen to what you say to yourself. What are your expectations of yourself? What do your doctor and other health-care professionals ask and expect of you? Being flexible is the goal—not being perfect. Be careful not to use judgmental phrases, such as I cheated today or I've been bad. All that you should expect of yourself is to do the best you can each day. And some days that is easier to do than others.

Diabetes health professionals now have more tools and strategies than ever before to help you manage your diabetes—from new oral medications for people with type II diabetes to medications that slow kidney disease and shorter-acting insulins to match the speed at which food turns to glucose. Try to find health professionals who accept what you will do and what you can't do. Work together to create a program that works for you. Honesty is still the best policy—for yourself and your diabetes team.

Get to know yourself

As we have said, the first step in changing behavior is to get to know yourself. For food and meal planning, that means learning what, where, when, and how much you eat during the day, at night, on the weekends, etc. At the end of chapters 3–10, you had an opportunity to get to know yourself better. From your answers, you see your strengths and the areas you need to make changes. Do not just read that section. After you've made a few changes, go back and ask yourself the questions again. Assess your new eating patterns, and decide your next step.

Self-assessment is key

You should keep records of blood glucose test results, the food you eat, physical activity, and medications. Talk to your health professional about what you need to record and when. Maybe you will decide that for the next 3 months you want to walk more. You should track the time you walk, the length of the walk, and the walk's effect on your blood glucose. Maybe during this time you don't need to keep food records, too. However, for good diabetes control, you need to test blood glucose daily and record the results.

Keep records your way

Keep records that work for you and give you the information you need. Bring these records when you visit your health-care provider to get feedback on your results. Records should be easy to use and in a form that can go with you. Maybe one of the following options will work for you:

▲ Use an appointment cal-
endar. Say that your
goal is to eat 5 servings
of fruits and vegetables
each day. In a corner of
each day's block, make a
mark for each serving of
fruit and vegetables that
you eat.

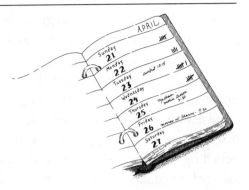

▲ Use the note section in the back of your calendar. Your food
record can include the date, time of meals and snacks, what
foods you ate, how they were prepared, and the quantity you
ate. You might note what food pyramid group the food is from.
This helps you see if you are eating by the pyramid.

▲ Design and carry a form in a separate notebook.

▲ Get a calendar specifically designed for keeping health records.

▲ Create a form on your computer. Maintain records on a disk
and print them out when you visit your health professional.

▲ Keep records on a hand-held computer calendar. Print them
out when you visit your health professional.

▲ Use the memory program in your blood glucose monitor.

▲ Use a record-keeping book provided by a diabetes supply company.

You need to find time to keep records. Are you an early bird?
Does it make sense to record yesterday's information early the next
morning? Or are you up late and have time then to update your
records? Are you forgetful and cannot remember what you eat
longer than an hour or two? You'll probably need to record information immediately.

Make records work for you

Use your records to see whether your current meal plan works and
to see what happens when you make changes in your regimen.
Bring your records when you visit your health-care providers. Talk
about patterns you've observed, for example, that your blood glucose is always higher than your target before dinner or that when

you drink fruit juice at the beginning of a meal, your blood glucose goes up quicker than when you eat a piece of fruit at the end of the meal.

Ask questions. For example, you see that, over the last few months, your blood glucose is higher 1 hour after dinner than it is all day long. What should you do about that? Ask for suggestions of how to fit in 3 fruit servings a day. Ask whether you should be recording anything else. For instance, you just record blood glucose before meals and it is between 80 and 160, yet your glycated hemoglobin is 8.4%. This shows that your average blood glucose is near 200. Perhaps you should check blood glucose 1 and 2 hours after meals to see how high it goes. Record keeping is an ongoing process. Think about what you want to find out and what changes you want to make.

Set your goals one step at a time

To manage diabetes, you may need to change the way you do things, to eat less fried food, eat breakfast every day, get more exercise, and so on. Don't try to make all these changes in one day. These habits were formed over years. Eating habits are particularly hard to change. This is why you need to set goals one at a time.

How do you choose which habit to change first? Choose one that you feel you can change easily. If you successfully change one habit, you're more likely to tackle the next eagerly. An easy change is the food you eat for nighttime snacks or simply switching from whole milk to skim. A more difficult change would be to start eating breakfast if you never have.

Ready, set goals

Each goal you set should
▲ be realistic
▲ be easy to achieve
▲ be specific
▲ have a short time frame
Here are a few examples:
1. You see that you eat breakfast on the run from a fast-food spot

or the cafeteria at work Monday through Friday. Your usual choices are a sausage biscuit, a bagel with a thick layer of regular cream cheese, or a mega muffin and a banana. You realize you have other choices.

Goal to change behavior:

For the next 2 months (*short time frame*), 2 days each week (*specific*) I will choose one of these healthier breakfasts: an English muffin with jelly and a small banana or a bagel with light or fat-free cream cheese with an orange or half grapefruit (*realistic and easy to achieve*).

2. You realize that you consume little or no milk or yogurt over the course of a week.

Goal to change behavior:

For the next month (*short time frame*), 3 days each week (*specific*) I will buy a carton of milk with my lunch or take a container of refrigerated nonfat fruited yogurt to eat as dessert (*realistic and easy to achieve*).

Now, it's your turn. Take a piece of paper and write a few goals based on what you discovered about your eating habits. Write your answers to the questions in the Get to Know Yourself sections of chapters 3–10.

Also, look at your recent food records, or think about what you eat day in and day out. Make your goals easy to reach. Keep your goals handy so you can see them frequently—in your calendar, on the refrigerator, or on your night table. At the end of the time frame you set, answer these questions.

▲ Did I meet my goals?

▲ If not, why not? Were they unrealistic?

▲ Was the time frame too long?

If the answers are yes, then make the goals easier to accomplish, or choose another goal that you can achieve. If you met your goals, pat yourself on the back!

Step by step you change

A new habit that you practice day after day and month after month becomes part of you. For instance, you always remember to stick a piece of fruit in your briefcase before you leave home in the morning and eat it during the afternoon. Or you automatically choose a garden salad with light dressing at a fast-food restaurant rather than french fries. Or you feel sluggish if you do not get your 20-minute after-lunch walk at least 3 days a week.

Now you know

▲ The importance of honesty to yourself and your health-care providers.

▲ If you want to make behavior changes, you need to learn about your current habits.

▲ The importance of record keeping for good diabetes management.

▲ The four parts of a goal and how to set them.

Scenario

Meet Charles. Charles now officially has diabetes. About 7 years ago, when he was 67, his doctor told him he had "borderline diabetes." His doctor told Charles to take one pill in the morning to help lower his blood glucose and to stay away from sweets. At that time Charles was 25 pounds overweight. His doctor also said it would be a good idea to take off a few pounds. Charles' doctor did not recommend that he see a dietitian or get any other education about diabetes. He did send Charles to an ophthalmologist (eye doctor).

Charles went back to see his doctor every six months or so. A week before he went, he would eat fewer sweets and try to take off a few pounds by eating smaller portions. When his doctor checked his fasting blood glucose, it was never much above 160 mg/dl. Two years ago Charles was having some troublesome symptoms—feeling tired, urinating a lot, and seeing spots in his eyes. He went back to his doctor. His doctor increased his medication and advised him again to limit sweets and to take off a few of his extra (now 30) pounds. This time he recommended that Charles see a dietitian to help him with his weight and blood glucose control. He also recommended that Charles go back to the ophthalmologist because he suspected that Charles had eye damage due to many years of uncontrolled diabetes.

Charles went to the eye doctor and found that he did have some vision problems due to diabetes. The eye doctor recommended that Charles get his blood glucose in control and take his diabetes seriously. Charles also went to see the dietitian.

Charles was scared about the damage that diabetes was doing to his eyes, so he was ready to be honest and to make some changes. When the dietitian asked what he usually eats, as much as he hated to, he told the truth. He admitted he eats sweets at least once a day and fried foods several times a week, even though he knows those foods aren't healthy for him.

Charles says he isn't much for fruits and vegetables but tries to eat one of each a day. The dietitian tells him he has several changes to make to eat healthier, control blood glucose, and help stop the damage high blood glucose is doing. She shows Charles the diabetes food pyramid to help him understand what he should eat.

They set a few healthy eating goals based on the food pyramid and what Charles is willing to do. He will try to eat at least 2 servings of fruit and 2 servings of vegetables each day. He will try to limit sweets to 4 days a week and fried foods to once a week, because sweets and fried foods are so high in fat and calories.

The RD noted how important exercise is. Charles will try to walk for 20 minutes, 3 times a week. He will also keep food records during 3 days of each week, 2 weekdays and 1 weekend day. She gave him a form to record the food he eats.

She also encouraged Charles to test his blood glucose. Charles hates doing this but he agreed to do it once a day. They agreed on a schedule to test at different times once a day to give him a sense of what his blood glucose is during the day. She gave him a book to record blood glucose levels, the time he does the test, his medication, and any comments or questions he has about the blood glucose results. Charles will come back in about a month to discuss his progress and to see if he is ready to set more goals to get better control of his diabetes.

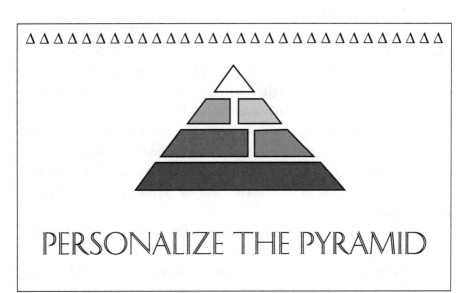

CHAPTER 13

PERSONALIZE THE PYRAMID

What you will learn

▲ How to use the pyramid to set your goals for healthy eating.

▲ How many calories you need to eat.

▲ How many servings you should eat from each food group.

▲ What are RDAs, USRDAs, and RDIs and how to use them.

▲ Good foods to eat for vitamins and minerals.

Create your pyramid

Put the pyramid to work for you. You'll eat servings from each of the five food groups every day. The amount of fats, sweets, and alcohol you can include in your meal plan depends on the number of calories that you need.

How many calories should you eat?

Look at the chart on page 147. If you are a small woman (under 5'4"), then 1400 calories is a good place to start. If you want to lose weight, 1200 calories might be enough. If you are a man younger than 50 years and you have a physically demanding job or exercise a lot, 2800 calories is your target.

Aim for a range

The actual number of calories you eat on any one day will not be exactly 1400 or 2800. That is why the calorie range is given. The lower number in the calorie range applies if you eat about 20% of daily calories as fat. The higher number in the calorie range applies if you eat about 40% of daily calories as fat.

The exact number of calories you eat each day greatly depends on the fat content of the foods you choose. Balance is important. If you eat some higher-fat choices one day, choose lower-fat choices the next. Over time, your calories will be within the ranges given on the chart.

You do not need to aim for a specific calorie range. Instead, focus your goals on the principles of the food pyramid—eat more grains, fruit, and vegetables, and eat fewer meats, fats, and sweets. Your calories will automatically come down.

How many servings for you?

Once you have your calorie range, look at the number of servings you need from each food group. For example, for 1600 calories, you need

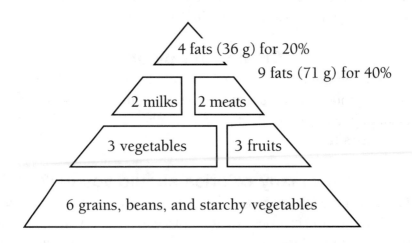

Servings per day

Calorie level Calorie range†	Weight loss* women About 1200 1200–1500	Many older women About 1400 1300–1600	Women, older adults About 1600 1400–1700	Larger women, older men About 1800 1600–1900	Children, teen girls, active women, most men About 2200 1800–2300	Teen boys, active men About 2800 2200–2800
Grains, beans, and starchy vegetables	6	6	6	7	9	11
Vegetables	3	3	3	4	4	5
Fruits	3	3	3	3	3	4
Milk‡	2	2	2–3	2–3	2–3	2–3
Meats	2 (4 oz)	2 (4 oz)	2 (5 oz)	2 (5 oz)	2 (6 oz)	3 (7 oz)
Fats g/servings						
20%	27/2	31/4	36/4	40/5	49/6	62/8
40%	53/5	62/8	71/9	80/11	98/13	124/18

*Some older women and men who are small and sedentary may need to eat 1200 calories to lose weight. At 1200 calories, you may need a vitamin and mineral supplement. If you burn calories with physical activity, you can eat more.

†Lower number is based on 20% fat, 2 servings of skim milk, and low-fat food choices; higher number is based on 40% fat, 3 servings of skim milk, and higher-fat food choices.

‡Teenagers, young adults to age 24, and women who are pregnant or breastfeeding need 1200 mg of calcium each day. That equals about 4 servings of milk and yogurt. Eating skim and nonfat milk and yogurt will keep fat grams and calories lower.

Divide calories into meals and snacks

After you know the total number of servings you need from each food group, divide these servings among your meals and snacks. Think about how much and what type of food to eat at each one. These decisions are based on many factors. Here are a few:

▲ What foods you enjoy and when.

▲ Your diabetes medication schedule.

▲ How much you like to eat at different meals and snacks.

▲ Your need or desire to include snacks.

▲ Your need to be careful with the amount of nutrients you eat due to other diseases, for example, sodium and blood pressure or saturated fat and high cholesterol.

▲ How often you eat meals away from home, when, and what types of foods.

▲ Whether you take vitamin and mineral supplements.

▲ Your weight history and attempts to lose weight (if you are overweight).

▲ Your exercise habits: times of day you exercise, what you do, and for how long.

▲ Your life schedule: if you work, your work hours, how your weekdays vary from weekends, and other events in your schedule to consider.

Work with a dietitian. Your answers to the above questions will help the dietitian create a meal plan just for you.

Learn by example

Here are a few examples to help you see how to plan meals and snacks by using the pyramid. The examples include foods you prepare at home, recipes, convenience foods, fast foods, and other restaurant foods. The nutrients in each menu are given. You don't have to eat *exactly* the recommended amounts every day. It is most important to eat a variety of foods over a few days. (For more meal and snack menu ideas, see the *Month of Meals* series I–V published by the American Diabetes Association.)

About 1200 calories

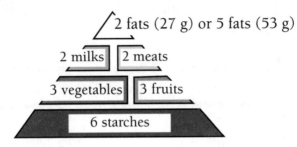

2 fats (27 g) or 5 fats (53 g)

2 milks   2 meats

3 vegetables   3 fruits

6 starches

Breakfast

1/2 cup oatmeal (cooked)	1 starch
1 Tbsp wheat germ, toasted	free food
4 dried apricot halves	1/2 fruit
1/2 cup skim milk	1/2 milk
1/2 cup cubes of papaya	1/2 fruit
1/2 cup plain nonfat yogurt	1/2 milk

Lunch

1/3 cup hummus*	1 starch
1/2 whole wheat pita pocket	1 starch
1/2 cup sliced cucumber	1/2 vegetable
1/3 cup alfalfa sprouts	1/2 vegetable
1 oz baked tortilla chips	1 starch
1 nectarine	1 fruit

Dinner

Salad bar	2–3 vegetables
1 1/2 cups romaine lettuce	
2 Tbsp chopped mushrooms	
1/3 cup canned beets	
1/3 cup three-bean salad	
2 Tbsp raisins	1 fruit
1 oz lean ham	1/2 meat
1 oz feta cheese	1/2 meat
2 Tbsp fat-free ranch salad dressing	free food
1 whole wheat dinner roll	1 starch

*Good source of protein. Takes place of 1 serving of meat and others.

Evening Snack

1 cup hot cocoa from mix	1 milk
3 gingersnaps	1 starch

Nutrition Facts	
Calories 1252	
Total fat 26g	18% of calories
Saturated 8.5g	
Monounsaturated 8g	
Cholesterol 47mg	
Sodium 2400mg	
Total carbohydrate 21g	65% of calories
Dietary fiber 15g	
Sugars 41g	
Protein 54g	17% of calories
Vitamin A 659 RE* •	Vitamin C 82mg
Calcium 757mg •	Iron 11mg
*RE is retinol equivalent	

About 1400 calories

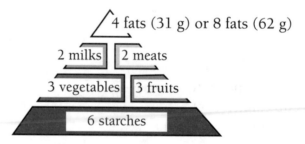

4 fats (31 g) or 8 fats (62 g)

2 milks | 2 meats

3 vegetables | 3 fruits

6 starches

Breakfast

1 cup Cheerios cereal	1 starch
1/2 cup All Bran cereal	1 starch
3/4 cup blueberries	1 fruit
1 cup skim milk	1 milk

Lunch

6 garlic melba toasts (round)	1 starch
2 oz swiss cheese	1 meat
1/2 cup (4 oz) nonfat fruited yogurt	
with aspartame	1/2 milk
1 kiwi fruit	1 fruit

Dinner

Chicken, rice, and vegetables	1 meat, 2 starches,
frozen entree	2 vegetables
Salad	2 vegetables
1 cup romaine lettuce	
1/2 sliced red pepper	
1/4 cup sliced canned beets	
1 Tbsp blue cheese dressing (regular)	5 g fat
1 Tbsp balsamic vinegar	free food

Evening Snack

1 fresh peach, sliced	1 fruit
1/4 cup Grape-Nuts	1 starch
1/2 cup nonfat sugar-free yogurt	1/2 milk

Nutrition Facts	
Calories 1350	
Total fat 31g	20% of calories
Saturated 13g	
Monounsaturated 7g	
Cholesterol 90mg	
Sodium 2160mg	
Total carbohydrate 206g	61% of calories
Dietary fiber 28g	
Sugars 61g	
Protein 78g	23% of calories
Vitamin A 1600 RE • Vitamin C 215mg	
Calcium 1302mg • Iron 21mg	

About 1600 calories

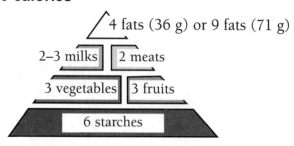

4 fats (36 g) or 9 fats (71 g)

2–3 milks | 2 meats

3 vegetables | 3 fruits

6 starches

Breakfast

1 bagel (small), sesame	2 starches
2 Tbsp cream cheese, fat free	free food, 2 servings
2 tsp low-sugar jam	free
1 small banana (4 oz)	1 fruit

Lunch

Tuna salad

2 oz tuna, water-packed	1 meat
1 Tbsp of mayonnaise, low fat	5 g fat
2 Tbsp low-fat cottage cheese	free
2 Tbsp diced celery	vegetable
1 Tbsp diced onions	vegetable
2 slices whole wheat bread	2 starches
1 cup raw or blanched broccoli	1 vegetable
1 cup skim milk	1 milk
1 small apple	1 fruit

Afternoon Snack

1 cup/8 oz nonfat fruited yogurt	1 milk

Dinner

Oriental stir-fry fish and vegetables	1 meat, 2 vegetables
2/3 cup basmati rice	2 starches

Evening Snack

Fruit dessert

1/3 cup sliced fresh pineapple	1/2 fruit
1/2 small sliced banana	1/2 fruit
1 Tbsp orange liqueur	free food
1/2 cup light ice cream	sweet

Nutrition Facts	
Calories 1624	
Total fat 36g	20% of calories
Saturated 8g	
Monounsaturated 10g	
Cholesterol 96mg	
Sodium 2056mg	
Total carbohydrate 244g	58% of calories
Dietary fiber 21g	
Sugars 97g	
Protein 88g	22% of calories
Vitamin A 449 RE • Vitamin C 125 mg	
Calcium 1070 mg • Iron 11 mg	

About 1800 calories

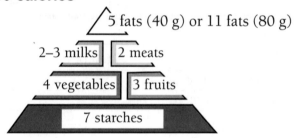

5 fats (40 g) or 11 fats (80 g)

2–3 milks | 2 meats

4 vegetables | 3 fruits

7 starches

Breakfast

Strawberry milkshake	1 milk, 1 fruit
1 slice whole wheat bread	1 starch
1 oz low-fat cheese	1/2 meat

Lunch

1 cup black bean soup	1 starch, 2 vegetables
4 whole wheat fat-free crackers	1 starch
2 oz canned salmon	1 meat
1 Tbsp mayonnaise, low fat	5 g fat
1/2 cup cubes jicama	1 vegetable
1 cup cubes cantaloupe	1 fruit

Dinner—at Mexican restaurant

12 oz beer, light	alcohol
Split order of combination fajitas	
2 flour tortillas	2 starches
1 1/2 oz grilled chicken	1/2 meat
1 1/2 oz grilled beef	1/2 meat
sautéed onions and peppers	1 vegetable
lettuce and tomato	1 vegetable
1/3 cup Mexican rice	1 starch
Flan (caramel custard)	sweet

Evening Snack

3 graham crackers	1 starch
3/4 cup blueberries	1 fruit
1 cup nonfat plain yogurt	1 milk

Nutrition Facts

Calories 1874		
Total fat 50g	26% of calories	
Saturated 14g		
Monounsaturated 18g		
Cholesterol 245mg		
Sodium 2928mg		
Total carbohydrate 245g	52% of calories	
Dietary fiber 19g		
Sugars 66g		
Protein 98g	22% of calories	
Vitamin A 2079 RE	•	Vitamin C 266mg
Calcium 1442mg	•	Iron 12mg
Alcohol 13g	5% of calories	

About 2200 calories

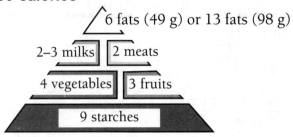

6 fats (49 g) or 13 fats (98 g)

2–3 milks | 2 meats

4 vegetables | 3 fruits

9 starches

Breakfast

1 egg	1/2 meat
1 whole English muffin	2 starches
1/4 cup stewed prunes	1 fruit
1 cup skim milk	1 milk

Lunch

1 1/4 lb fast food hamburger	2 starches, 1 meat
1 order small french fries	1 starch
2 Tbsp ketchup	free
1 garden salad	1 vegetable
2 Tbsp fat-free Italian dressing	free

Afternoon Snack

2 rice cakes	1 starch
2 Tbsp peanut butter	1/2 meat
1 1/2 dried figs	1 fruit

Dinner

1 cup turkey chili	1 starch, 1 vegetable, 1 meat
1 small baked potato	1 starch
1/2 cup blanched zucchini	1 vegetable
1/2 cup blanched green beans	1 vegetable
with 4 Tbsp fresh dill dip	1/4 milk

Evening Snack

3/4 cup bran flakes	1 starch
3/4 cup skim milk	3/4 milk
8 dried apricot halves	1 fruit

Nutrition Facts

Calories 2147			
Total fat 75g		30% of calories	
Saturated 19g			
Monounsaturated 27g			
Cholesterol 458mg			
Sodium 3100mg			
Total carbohydrate 296g		53% of calories	
Dietary fiber 30g			
Sugars 92g			
Protein 97g		17% of calories	
Vitamin A	1765 RE	•	Vitamin C 119mg
Calcium	1143mg	•	Iron 27mg
Alcohol	13g		5% of calories

About 2800 calories

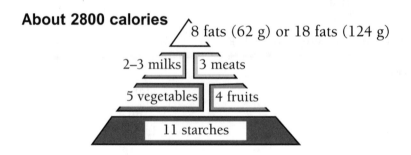

8 fats (62 g) or 18 fats (124 g)

2–3 milks | 3 meats

5 vegetables | 4 fruits

11 starches

Breakfast

3 frozen waffles	3 starches
2 Tbsp maple syrup	2 starches
2 tsp margarine	10 g fat
1/2 cup nonfat plain yogurt	1/2 milk
1 cup fruit: grapefruit, orange, apple, and banana	2 fruits

Morning Snack

1/3 cup dried apples	1 fruit
1/8 cup pecans	5 g fat

Lunch

1 slice pizza with mushrooms, peppers, and onions	3 starches, 1 vegetable, 1 meat
1 salad	1 vegetable
2 Tbsp Caesar salad dressing	10 g fat

Afternoon Snack

1 granola bar	1 starch
1 cup skim milk	1 milk

Dinner

6 oz white wine	
4 oz beef liver, cooked	2 meats
1/2 cup onions (with 1 tsp olive oil)	1 vegetable, 5 g fat
1 medium sweet potato	2 starches
1 cup steamed spinach with lemon	2 vegetables
1 whole wheat dinner roll	1 starch

Evening Snack

1 piece angel food cake	2 starches/sweet
1 cup frozen unsweetened strawberries	1 fruit
1/2 cup frozen yogurt	1 milk

Nutrition Facts	
Calories 2837	
Total fat 93g	30% of calories
Saturated 24g	
Monounsaturated 22 g	
Cholesterol 746mg	
Sodium 3200mg	
Total carbohydrate 375g	53% of calories
Dietary fiber 35g	
Sugars 112g	
Protein 118g	17% of calories
Vitamin A 18427RE •	Vitamin C 261mg
Calcium 2100mg •	Iron 28mg
Alcohol 16g	5% of calories

RDA

Recommended Daily Allowances (RDAs) are the amounts of essential nutrients—mainly vitamins and minerals—that all healthy people need. RDAs are revised about every 5 years by a group of scientists appointed by a United States government agency. RDAs are different for various age groups and phases of life. For instance, RDAs are different for pregnancy, childhood, and adolescents, because nutritional needs change during those times.

Are RDAs high enough?

The current RDAs are high enough to prevent vitamin deficiencies, such as scurvy from lack of vitamin C. However, some scientists believe that several RDAs are not high enough to prevent diseases such as cancer and heart disease. Scientists will research this question over the next few years.

USRDA

U.S. Recommended Daily Allowances (USRDAs) are one set of nutrient recommendations, regardless of age group or phase of life for programs such as food labels and standards for school lunches. USRDAs are actually the RDAs from 1968 for teenage boys. These are used because teenage boys have the highest RDAs.

The scientists who created the RDAs believe that when you eat a wide variety of healthy foods each day, especially enough servings of fruits, vegetables, and grains, you'll get the nutrients you need.

RDI

Reference Daily Intakes (RDIs) are the numbers used to find the Daily Values on food labels. Currently, RDIs are just another name for USRDAs. They were given a different name because new RDIs may be set in the future.

Fewer calories equal fewer nutrients

As your calories increase, it is easier to get all the nutrients you need. At lower calorie levels, say, less than 1400 calories, you have to try hard to eat a wide variety of foods. If you usually eat less than

1200 calories a day or you cannot eat a particular category of foods, consult with your doctor or dietitian about taking a vitamin and mineral supplement.

Antioxidants and diabetes

Antioxidants—vitamins E, A (beta-carotene), and C—do important work as scavengers, picking up free radicals in your body. Free radicals float around your body damaging cells. Antioxidants are like Pac-Man. They gobble up free radicals in the blood stream and whisk them out of the body.

Research shows a connection between free radicals, antioxidants, and diabetes. High blood glucose helps free radicals form in the body. And the free radicals seem to take part in some diabetes complications. Additional research is being done to check this. The most important advice right now is to eat the number of fruits and vegetables in your meal plan.

Top 10 by A B C

The following charts give you a list of the top 10 foods for certain vitamins and minerals. The chart lists the food, the serving, the pyramid group, and the amount of nutrient per serving. Use these lists to help you choose foods to meet your vitamin and mineral needs.

Vitamin A (USRDA 1000 RE [retinol equivalents])			
Food	Serving	Food Group	Vitamin A
Liver, beef, cooked	3 oz	Meat	8934
Liver, chicken, cooked	3 oz	Meat	5165
Sweet potato	1/2 cup	Starch	3682
Pumpkin, canned	3/4 cup	Fruit	2702
Salmon, cooked	3 oz	Meat	2826
Carrots, raw or cooked	1/2 cup	Vegetable	1970
Cantaloupe	1/3	Fruit	1565
Eel, cooked	3 oz	Meat	966
Squash, winter	1 cup	Starch	1435
Cereal, cold, whole grain	3/4 cup	Starch	855

Vitamin C (USRDA/RDI 60 mg)

Food	Serving	Food Group	Vitamin C (mg)
Grapefruit	1/2	Fruit	46
Orange	1	Fruit	70
Kiwi	1 whole	Fruit	75
Cantaloupe	1 cup	Fruit	31
Honeydew	1 cup	Fruit	42
Papaya	1/2 whole	Fruit	43
Strawberries	1 1/4 cups	Fruit	106
Apple juice	1/3 cup	Fruit	31
Green pepper	1 cup	Vegetable	60
Tomato soup	1 cup	Vegetable	66

Vitamin E (USRDA/RDI 30 IU or 10 mg)

Food	Serving	Food Group	Vitamin E (mg)
Salad dressing, regular and reduced calorie	1 Tbsp	Fat	2.7–7.5
Peanut butter	2 Tbsp	Fat	6.4
Sunflower seeds	1 Tbsp	Fat	4.7
Vegetable oils	1 tsp	Fat	2.6–4.7
Sweet potato	1/2 cup	Starch	7.6
Lima beans	2/3 cup	Starch	8.6
Cereal, cold, whole grain	3/4 cup	Starch	4.0–8.7
Whole wheat dinner roll, yeast	1 roll	Starch	3.8
Margarines	1 tsp	Fat	1.9–3.5
Nuts	6–10	Fat	0.9–3.6

Folic Acid (USRDA/RDI 0.4 mg)

Food	Serving	Food Group	Folic Acid (mg)
Liver, chicken	3 oz	Meat	650
Cereal, cold, bran type	1/2 cup	Starch	225
Liver, beef	3 oz	Meat	190
Beans (lentils, kidney, black, white)	1/2 cup	Starch	120–180

Food	Serving	Food Group	
Asparagus	1/2 cup	Vegetable	120
Cereal, cold, whole grain, flakes	3/4 cup	Starch	40–120
Spinach	1/2 cup	Vegetable	112
Lettuce, romaine	1 cup	Vegetable	80
Peas (black-eyed peas, split, green)	1/2 cup	Starch	50–80
Vegetables (artichoke, beets, brussel sprouts, collard and turnip greens)	1/2 cup	Vegetable	50–65

Calcium (USRDA 1000 mg)

Food	Serving	Food Group	Calcium (mg)
Milk, skim and 1% fat	1 cup	Milk	300–350
Buttermilk (nonfat)	1 cup	Milk	285
Chocolate milk, 1% fat	1 cup	Milk	285
Yogurt, refrigerated	1 cup	Milk	250–350
Cheese, hard (cheddar, swiss, processed American)	1 oz	Meat	175–250
regular, reduced calorie	1 oz	Meat	175–250
Feta cheese	1 oz	Meat	145
Custard/Pudding, homemade	1/2 cup	Sweet	200–250
mix or ready to eat	1/2 cup	Sweet	110–150
Salmon, canned with bones	3 oz	Meat	180–210
Greens, collards, kale, spinach, turnips	1/2 cup	Vegetable	90–180
Figs, fresh or dried	2 med.	Fruit	145

Iron (USRDA/RDI 18 mg)

Food	Serving	Food Group	Iron (mg)
Oysters, cooked	3 oz	Meat	9
Liver, beef or chicken	3 oz	Meat	7
Clams, cooked	3 oz	Meat	15
Cereal, cold, whole grain, flakes	3/4 cup	Starch	5–10

Soybeans, boiled	1/2 cup	Meat	7
Spinach	1/2 cup	Vegetable	4
Shrimp, cooked	3 oz	Meat	3
Tofu	1/2 cup	Meat	2
Apricots	8 halves	Fruit	2

Magnesium (USRDA 400 mg)

Food	Serving	Food Group	Magnesium (mg)
Fish, white type	3 oz	Meat	40–90
Oysters, cooked	3 oz	Meat	40–90
Wheat germ	3 Tbsp	Starch	57
Greens (beet, collard, spinach, swiss chard)	1/2 cup	Vegetable	57
Beans (black-eyed peas, lima and navy)	1/2 cup	Starch	50
Millet, cooked	1/2 cup	Starch	50
Peanut butter	2 Tbsp	Meat/fat	50
Okra	1/2 cup	Vegetable	46
Yogurt, plain, nonfat	1 cup	Milk	43
Nuts (brazil, cashews, hazel)	1/8 cup	Fat	40

Now you know

▲ The range of calories you need to eat based on your sex, physical activity, diabetes, and nutrition goals.

▲ The number of servings to eat from each food group.

▲ What to consider when you plan how to divide your servings into meals and snacks.

▲ How to plan 1-day menus with convenience foods, fast foods, other restaurant foods, and recipes.

▲ The meaning of RDAs, USRDAs, and RDIs and how to use them.

▲ The top 10 sources of foods for many vitamins and minerals.

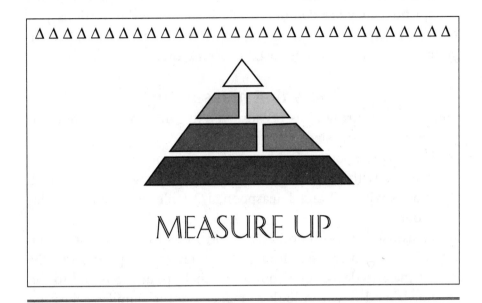

CHAPTER 14

MEASURE UP

What you will learn

▲ Accurate measurement of foods makes or breaks diabetes and weight control.

▲ Portion control is mastered with continued practice.

▲ The tools for portion control.

▲ Tips and tricks to eat the correct portion sizes.

Serving size counts

It just doesn't seem possible that an extra half cup of carrots or another teaspoon of margarine makes a big difference. But they do, for your weight and blood glucose control. You may overeat by 200, 300, or 400 calories each day. Perhaps you grab a piece of fresh fruit that is larger than the serving size. Or you have an extra one-third cup of pasta or an extra ounce of chicken. You might think it's OK because these foods are "healthy." But these add enough calories to make a difference in weight loss or gain and blood glucose control.

Servings have grown

Years ago, jumbo orders of french fries, 32-oz servings of soda, triple decker hamburgers, or all-you-can-eat buffets were unheard of, but now they are commonplace. If these are the portions you see every day, you will need to adjust your "eyeballs." Measure your servings until you get used to seeing them.

Tools that measure up

You need measuring tools because you're going to use them often to measure serving sizes.

▲ **Measuring spoons**: Don't use the teaspoons and tablespoons you eat with to measure servings. Have a set of measuring spoons with 1/2 and 1 teaspoon, 1/2 tablespoon, and 1 table-spoon.

▲ **Measuring cup—liquids**: A liquid measuring cup should be clear so you can see through it. To measure liquids correctly, set the cup down on a counter or shelf, pour the liquid to the line, bend down to look to make sure the liquid reaches the line. Don't hold the cup up in the air to check.

▲ **Measuring cup—solids**: Use the measuring cup equal to what you want, and fill it to the top. Level it with a flat knife edge to get rid of any excess.

▲ **Food scale**: It's good to have at least an inexpensive ($5–10) food scale, particularly for measuring foods you measure in ounces, like meat, fish, or cheese.

▲ **Eyeballs**: Well-trained and honest eyeballs are your best mea-suring tool because they are always with you.

Tricks to measure by

Put these strategies to work for successful portion control.

▲ When you purchase fresh produce (fruit, vegetables, and starches) use the food scales in the produce area. Weigh indi-vidual pieces of fruit. This will give you an idea of what a 4-oz banana, 6 1/2-oz orange, or 3 1/2-oz kiwi looks like. Use a food scale at home to recheck the weight.

▲ It is easy to go overboard with protein foods, especially meat, poultry, and cheese; because one more ounce does not look like much. However, it is another 35–100 calories for each ounce.

When you buy a package of cheese or anything you buy by the ounce, look at the ounces on the label. Then visualize what 1, 2, or 3 ounces look like.

▲ For a visual image, 3 oz of cooked meat is about the size of a deck of cards or the palm of your hand.

▲ At home, use the same size plates, glasses, and bowls. This helps you judge correct portions without having to use measuring tools every time. For instance, use the same glass for milk. Measure it out in a measuring cup once or twice. Pour it into the glass. See where that quantity reaches. Mark it if you want with an indelible marker or piece of masking tape. Then see how much room 1 cup of pasta takes on a dinner plate, one-half cup of hot oatmeal in a bowl, and so on. Keep these pictures in your mind.

▲ When you can eyeball honestly, you don't have to weigh and measure everything. It is wise to do so from time to time, perhaps once a week, just to refresh your mental pictures.

▲ Quiz yourself occasionally. Measure dry cereal, pasta, or rice in the dish you eat it in. Put it into a measuring cup. Is the serving correct? If not, readjust your mental picture, and measure in a measuring cup for awhile.

The food labels help

The serving size on the Nutrition Facts label on packaged foods will help you. Serving sizes are regulated by the FDA. That means that 1 serving of dry cereal is always 30 g or about 1 oz for all dry cereals on the market. In addition, manufacturers must also give you the serving in common household terms. For example, 3/4 cup cereal, 1 slice of bread, or 2 cookies. If you usually eat a larger quantity of that food, perhaps your servings are too large, or you're really having 2 servings.

When dining out

Getting correct servings can be a challenge in restaurants. Servings are usually too big. You can deal with large servings by ordering half-portions of pasta, splitting an entree, or taking home the excess in a doggie bag. If you weigh and measure foods at home, your eyeballs are your best defense. The more you can visualize the proper serving, the easier it is to follow your meal plan. One reminder about meats in restaurants. If they tell you a portion on the menu, it is a raw quantity, such as a quarter-pound hot dog or 12-oz rib eye steak. Apply the rule of thumb about converting from raw to cooked. (See page 67.)

Now you know

▲ It is important to weigh and measure foods often to eat the correct portion.

▲ Weighing and measuring foods can help you achieve your diabetes and weight goals.

▲ The tools you should have at home to weigh and measure foods are measuring spoons, measuring cups (liquid and solid), and a food scale.

▲ How to measure portions at the supermarket, in restaurants, and at home to help you eat correct portions.

Scenario

Meet Sarah. She learned the hard way that portion control matters. Sarah first found out her blood glucose was high at a health fair sponsored by her employer. It was 324 mg/dl. She quickly made an appointment to see her doctor to report her high blood glucose and to see whether she has diabetes. Indeed, her fasting blood glucose was 295 mg/dl one morning and 318 mg/dl soon after breakfast. Her doctor said she clearly has diabetes.

Sarah is about 35 pounds overweight, so her doctor suggested that she visit with a dietitian to develop a weight loss plan. Her doctor said she could probably control her diabetes, at least for the next several years, with exercise and weight loss. Sarah knew she had some hard work ahead. She made an appointment to see a dietitian.

Sarah left the dietitian's office with information about how to use the Diabetes Food Pyramid for meal planning. The dietitian said Sarah should aim for 1200–1400 calories a day and spread her servings out into three meals and one snack at night:

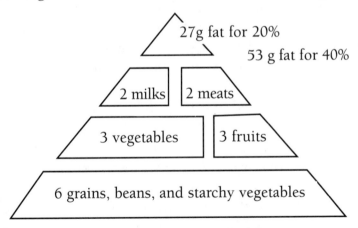

Sarah returned several weeks later and was frustrated by her lack of weight loss. She and the dietitian talked about weighing and measuring portions. Sarah said that when it came to fruits, vegetables, and starches, she depends on her eyeballs to judge portions. Sarah thought that a little extra here and there of these "healthy" foods would not add up to many calories. The dietitian said it is those extras that can make the difference, especially when you're trying to lose weight. The dietitian showed Sarah this convincing example:

–an extra 1/4 cup of hot oatmeal = 40+ calories
–a banana that is 6 oz rather than 4 oz = 30+ calories
–an apple that is 6 oz rather than 4 oz = 30+ calories
–an extra 1/4 cup of green peas = 40+ calories
–an extra 1/2 cup of asparagus = 25+ calories
–1 extra tsp canola oil in a salad = 45+ calories

These few extras add up to 190 calories over just 1 day. If that happens day after day, it can mean not achieving weight loss and good blood glucose control. Therefore, they talked about the tools Sarah needs to weigh and measure her foods at home, as well as some strategies for the supermarket and restaurants.

Sarah was determined to see the needle on the scale go down at her next visit to the dietitian. She dug out her measuring cups, teaspoons, and dusty old food scale. When gathering her apples, oranges, bananas along with potatoes and tomatoes for the week, she put them one by one on the food scale. Sure enough, the apples, potatoes, and bananas were several ounces larger than the food pyramid serving. With oranges and tomatoes she was on the mark.

When Sarah wanted to eat her usual breakfast of dry cereal, rather than pouring it straight into the bowl, she took the time to pour it into the measuring cup first. Yes, she was heavy handed with cereal. That was also true for meats—a half ounce here and an ounce there. As for fats, even though she uses the reduced-calorie and fat-free varieties of mayonnaise, cream cheese, and salad dressing, she was surprised when she read the Nutrition Facts to see how much her servings went over the line and how many calories that added. Sarah was now convinced—watching the serving size matters. And the best proof? When Sarah saw the dietitian a month later, she'd lost 2 pounds.

CHAPTER 15

PLANNING: A MUST FROM MENU TO MARKET TO TABLE

What you will learn

▲ Why planning is a key to healthier eating.

▲ Why planning, from menu to market to table, gives you more time and money in your pocket.

▲ Steps to take before you go to the supermarket.

▲ Tactics for stocking your kitchen to eat pyramid style.

▲ How to tackle the supermarket aisles.

Catch-as-catch-can costs

Believe it or not, a catch-as-catch-can eating style can cost you in several ways. First, it costs healthwise. If you grab a fast-food meal here and a convenience food there, you usually end up eating fewer fruits, vegetables, and whole grains and more fat, sweets, and meats. That turns the pyramid upside down. You want to plan ahead so that you won't make food decisions when you are hungry.

Second, it costs you time. For example, if you have foods ready at home for quick dinners—a frozen pizza with salad, an extra portion of last night's dinner, or an individual portion of frozen leftovers to microwave—you can have a good meal on the table in no time.

Third, it costs you dollars. If you buy food at convenience stores, eat in restaurants, order foods to go, or cruise through fast-food drive-in windows, your money goes quickly. You save when you buy food from the supermarket or farmer's market. If you invest the time to plan, the investment pays off—from menu planning, to shopping, to cooking, to eating. Remember, you spend time in the beginning to save time in the end.

Ready to plan

Set aside time to plan. It just takes a few minutes. Figure out a convenient time—perhaps, early morning while sipping your morning beverage, late at night while winding down, or on a Sunday after the paper is read. Keep a notepad by your bedside, in the kitchen, in the family room, or in the car—any place you might get menu planning ideas. Find what works best for you.

Link menus to market

What will your meals and snacks be for this week? What foods do you need to have on hand for breakfasts, lunches, dinners, and snacks? How about beverages? Your food plan helps you create your shopping list, so the more detail, the better. For instance, if one of your goals is to eat more fruit, you need to plan when you will eat it and what you will eat. If your goal is 2 servings of fruit a day and you try to eat one at breakfast, then you want another to carry in your brown-bag lunch. If that is your plan and you shop once a week, how much fresh fruit, canned fruit, or dried fruit do you need to buy? Ask yourself questions like these:

▲ What will I eat for breakfast?

▲ How many frozen entrees do I want for the week?

▲ What recipe will I prepare, and is it easy to cook a double batch for leftovers?

▲ What food will I take to work?

Develop your shopping list as you plan meals and snacks. Once you get used to doing it, planning will become second nature. It will help you cut back on your trips to the supermarket. If you want to make a certain recipe, read it. What ingredients do you have? What ingredients do you need? Next, take stock of the foods you want to have in the freezer, refrigerator, and pantry. For instance, your list might include frozen or canned vegetables, tuna, mayonnaise, sauces, and spices. Know what foods you have on hand and what has been finished off. Get in the habit of keeping a shopping list going. Keep a piece of paper on a bulletin board or refrigerator. As soon as you empty something and you want to replace it, write it on your list.

How to take stock

You can develop shopping lists by the places you store food—freezer, refrigerator, and pantry. For each, follow the food pyramid group order—grains, beans, and starchy vegetables; vegetables; fruit; and so on. Add two columns, quantity "at home" and "to buy," to help you take inventory and create your shopping list at the same time (see the example below).

You don't need to rewrite the list every week. Create your list and make copies. Or put the list on your computer and print it out. Add or subtract items as you find foods you enjoy or ones that the family doesn't. Take the list to the supermarket, and let it guide you. (This is how they do it in restaurants!)

Grains, beans, starchy vegetables	At Home	To Buy
Freezer:		
corn	0	1
green peas	1	0
whole wheat tortillas	1/2	1
Refrigerator:		
whole wheat bread	1/4 loaf	1
bagels	3	6
squash	0	1 acorn
potatoes—baking	2	4
potatoes—red	3	1 bag

Grains, beans, starchy vegetables	At Home	To Buy
Pantry:		
whole grain crackers	1/3 box	1 box
beans and peas		
lentils, dry	0	0
white beans, dry	1/2 bag	0
canned beans		
kidney beans, canned	0	1
refried beans, canned	1	2

Fix quick and easy favorites

Find ten quick and easy recipes that you and your family enjoy. Try to always have ingredients for five of them on hand. Use this checklist to see if your recipes really are quick and easy.

▲ A limit of 5–8 ingredients

▲ Ingredients are easy to find and easy to keep on hand

▲ Easy to fix (may take some time to cook like soup or stew, but makes good leftovers)

▲ Follows the food pyramid (heavy on starches and vegetables, light on protein)

▲ You can make it on the weekend, in an evening, or in a few spare minutes

▲ Everyone in the family enjoys it

▲ Stores well as leftovers

▲ Travels well as a brown bag lunch

Next stop to shop

You have planned meals and snacks, done inventory, and created your shopping list, now you are ready to shop. Few people relish this trip. Supermarkets keep getting larger. There are endless aisles, nutrition information, long ingredient lists, and even longer lines at the checkout. Just tell yourself you are a modern day hunter and gatherer. This really is the most important thing you do. Try these tactics to save time and money.

▲ Shop at the same market. If you know where things are, you get through faster. Ask for help as soon as you need it. Generally, the employees can save you time and energy.

▲ Shop as seldom as you can. Your shopping frequency depends on your family's size, the amount of fresh produce you buy, how much you can carry, etc.

▲ Go to the market when it is not crowded. Many are open 24 hours a day.

▲ Shop once. Try to find one place where you buy almost everything.

▲ An empty stomach means a fuller shopping cart. Try not to shop when you are hungry.

▲ Let your shopping list be your guide.

▲ Do not retrace your footsteps. Get everything you need in each section and move to the next.

▲ Remember, the healthiest foods are usually around the edges—fruits and vegetables on one wall, meats, poultry down another, and dairy foods along another wall.

▲ Do not walk every aisle. If you know you do not need items on a particular aisle, move on to the next, especially if there are aisles with foods you are better off leaving behind.

▲ Buy the same foods week after week that satisfy your taste buds and nutrition needs. Then you don't spend too much time reading food labels. Watch for bargains and new foods. Once in a while, read a label or two. Variety is good.

▲ Read food labels to make sure you know what you're buying and that the food fits into your meal plan.

Now you know

▲ How planning helps you know what you will eat and what to buy in the supermarket.

▲ How to organize your shopping list and shopping journey.

▲ How to save time, steps, and dollars in the supermarket.

Scenario

Meet Leo. He has had type I diabetes half his life. He is 44 years old and works as an auto mechanic. Leo lives alone. He takes two shots of insulin a day, tests his blood glucose one or two times a day, and manages to keep his weight steady, probably because he is so active at work.

Leo has high blood pressure. He needs to limit the amount of sodium in his food. Leo's doctor discussed with Leo how high blood pressure can affect eyes and kidneys. He suggested that Leo visit the dietitian. He and the RD discussed his diabetes control and meal planning. Leo was honest and talked about the problems with his meal plan. Leo needs a lot of food—he's 6'2" and very active—but the foods he chooses are not always the healthiest.

Some days he eats a healthy breakfast, but other days, he gets a fast-food sausage biscuit or English muffin with egg, cheese, and ham. He takes lunch to work a few days—several sandwiches of ham, bologna, or salami. He buys potato or corn chips and a fruit drink at the job. Two nights a week, dinner is a frozen dinner; other nights, it is a home-cooked meal with a meat, starches, and vegetables. He orders in pizza with pepperoni and extra cheese once a week, and he eats one or two dinners out.

The RD focused on the high-sodium foods Leo eats. She listed the major ones—cold cuts, canned soup, many convenience foods, and cheese. Foods very low in sodium, she said, are the very healthy foods—grains, fruits, and vegetables.

Leo said he shops irregularly and keeps little food in the house. That is one reason he ends up at restaurants or ordering pizza. The RD suggested that Leo plan meals and snacks for the week, put together a shopping list, shop, and start the week with a full kitchen. Leo was willing to try this.

The RD gave Leo a few quick recipes to try—vegetable beef stew; bean and barley soup; and chicken, rice, and broccoli casserole. They talked about lower-sodium choices for breakfast and lunch and using spices rather than the salt shaker.

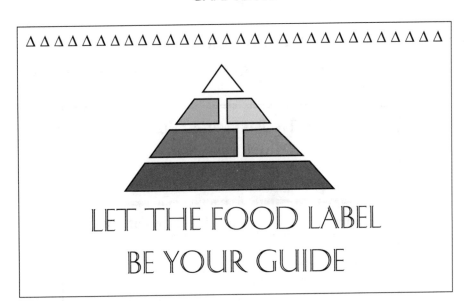

CHAPTER 16

LET THE FOOD LABEL BE YOUR GUIDE

What you will learn

▲ What foods must have nutrition labeling.

▲ What's on the food label and Nutrition Facts panel.

▲ How the Nutrition Facts panel helps you make healthy decisions.

▲ Similarities and differences in serving sizes between the food label and the diabetes pyramid.

▲ What food label nutrition claims mean.

▲ Healthy eating guidelines to use in the supermarket.

What's got a label?

▲ Almost all packaged and processed foods. The exceptions are very small packages with no room on the panel; bulk foods like cereals or nuts sold from the barrels; foods with no nutrients, like coffee, tea, spices, and herbs.

▲ Fresh fruits and vegetables—20 of the most common fruits and vegetables. You'll find the information posted near the item in the produce area.

▲ Meat and poultry—45 of the most common cuts of meat and poultry.

▲ Seafood—the 20 most common seafoods.

What's on the label?

Let's look at a label from a frozen entree, bow tie pasta with chicken and vegetables.

	Bow Tie Pasta and Chicken		
A	**Nutrition Facts**		
B	Serving size 1 package (269g)		
C	**Servings per container 1**		
D	**Calories 270** **Calories from Fat 50**		K
	% Daily Value*		
E	**Total fat** 6g	9%	
	Saturated fat 1.5g	6%	
	Polyunsaturated fat 1.5g		
	Monounsaturated fat 2g		
F	**Cholesterol** 60mg	20%	M
G	**Sodium** 550mg	22%	
H	**Total carbohydrate** 34g	11%	
	Dietary fiber 5g	19%	
	Sugars 6g		
I	**Protein** 19g		
J	Vitamin A 50% • Vitamin C 25%		
	Calcium 8% • Iron 15%		

*Percent Daily Values are based on a 2000 calorie diet. Your daily values may be higher or lower depending on your calorie needs.   L

	Calories	2000	2500
Total fat	less than	65g	80g
Sat fat	less than	20g	25g
Cholesterol	less than	300mcg	300mcg
Sodium	less than	2400mg	2400mg
Total carbohydrate		300g	375g
Dietary fiber		25g	30g

A. Nutrition Facts about the food.

B. Serving size.

C. Servings per container. Nutrition information is for 1 serving. For example, this frozen entree contains 1 serving, so the nutrition information is for the whole package.

D. Calories and calories from fat in 1 serving.

E. Total fats is the total number of grams of fat in 1 serving. The only type of fat that must be listed is saturated fat.

F. Cholesterol is listed in milligrams.

G. Sodium is listed in milligrams.

H. Total carbohydrate is the total number of grams of carbohydrate in 1 serving. The grams of two types of carbohydrates—dietary fiber and sugars—are listed under total carbohydrate. (See pages 13–28 for more about carbohydrates.)

I. Protein is the grams of protein in 1 serving.

J. Vitamins and minerals. The percentage of the Recommended Daily Intake (RDI) in the food for two vitamins, A and C, and two minerals, calcium and iron, must be listed.

If a nutrition claim is made about a vitamin or mineral (in addition to vitamins A, C, calcium, and iron), the percentage of RDI in the food must be on the label. For example, if a manufacturer states "one serving provides the day's need for B vitamins," they must include nutrition information for all the B vitamins. Manufacturers can list the nutrition content for more vitamins and minerals if they want to.

K. Percent Daily Values message.

L. The daily values are the amounts of each nutrient that a person who eats 2000 calories a day needs. It's like a mini–meal plan on the label. Larger packages also have the daily values for 2500 calories a day. Two thousand calories is used because it is an average calorie level for adults, but it may be high for you. Read more about daily values on pages 180–81.

M. % Daily Values for total fat, saturated fat, cholesterol, sodium, total carbohydrate, and dietary fiber are listed to the right of each nutrient. These numbers tell you what percentage of the daily value is in 1 serving of the food. (The asterisk by % Daily

Value refers you to K and L.) The rule of thumb: If it's 5% or less, it doesn't give you much of that nutrient. If it's 20% or more, it gives you enough of that nutrient to be important to your meal plan.

Other items you might see on the package:

Ingredients in the food are listed in descending order by weight. There are only tiny amounts of those ingredients that are at the end of the list.

Nutrition claim: If a nutrition claim is made, information about that claim must be given. In this example, the nutrition claim is low fat.

Calories per gram: Some longer labels tell you that fat has 9 calories per gram, carbohydrate has 4, and protein has 4.

Serving sizes get real

Standard serving sizes were developed for more than 100 foods. These servings are close to a typical serving. The serving size must also be given in household measures, such as cup, tablespoon, or the number of items, so you can picture it. For example, the serving size on a cracker label might read 15 crackers (28 g/1 oz).

Serving sizes not always a match

The standard serving size on food products may or may not be the same as those in the Diabetes Food Pyramid. What you need to do is compare the serving size on the label with the pyramid serving size. Check the chart on the next page for some examples. Some are the same and some are different.

If the serving sizes are the same, then it is easy to use the nutrition information. If different, you need to do some math. For example, you are reading the label from regular margarine and the serving size is 1 Tbsp. But 1 tsp is the pyramid serving size. To get nutrient information for 1 tsp, you need to divide the numbers on the label by 3 because there are 3 tsp in 1 Tbsp.

Comparison of Food Serving Sizes

Food	Food label serving	Food pyramid serving
Refrigerated yogurt (plain, nonfat)	1 cup	1 cup
Ice cream (light or frozen yogurt)	1/2 cup	1/2 cup
Dry cereal	30 g/oz	30 g/oz
Salad dressing (reduced calorie)	2 Tbsp	2 Tbsp
Butter or margarine (regular stick)	1 Tbsp	1 tsp
Fruit juice	8 oz	1/3–1/2 cup
Salad dressing (regular)	2 Tbsp	1 Tbsp

Play the numbers with fats

The new food label gives you important information about fats.

Calories from fat: This number tells you how many of the calories in the food are from fat. This is helpful information, but you don't have to limit yourself to foods that have 30% fat. Thirty percent is the guideline for the whole day—30% of all the calories you eat in 1 day.

One food you buy, such as canned peaches, will have zero calories from fat, but salad dressing might have 80% of calories from fat (because it is mainly fat). Does that mean you should not buy the salad dressing? No, you just balance that high-fat food by choosing other foods that are low in fat to round out the meals for that day.

To find the calories from fat for the whole day, add up all the calories you've eaten. Add up all the grams of fat that you've eaten that day. Multiply the grams of fat by 9 (each gram of fat has 9 calories) to see how many calories you got from fat. Divide the fat calories by the total calories for the day to see what percentage of total calories is from fat (600/2000 = 0.30 or 30%).

179

Total fat grams: This is the total grams of fat in 1 serving. Your meal plan tells you how many grams of fat to eat each day. You just need to add up the grams of fat in each food that you eat during the day.

Grams of saturated, polyunsaturated, and monounsaturated fat: These numbers help you see what types of fat the total grams of fat come from. Remember, you want to keep saturated fat down and monounsaturated fat up. Saturated fat is on almost every label.

Cholesterol: The cholesterol recommendation is 300 mg or less for everyone, so the daily value fits you no matter what your calorie range. The same is true for sodium.

While it is important to count fat grams, don't forget that calories count, too. Words like fat free or sugar free do not mean calorie free.

Get personal with daily values

The Daily Values on food labels given in grams and percentage are for a person eating 2000 calories a day. If you eat more or fewer calories, then your personal daily values will be different from those on the label. Ask your dietitian to help you figure out your own daily values. You can jot them down and carry them with you to the market and restaurants to make it easier to decide whether a food fits your meal plan.

How to use your daily values

Use this general rule: When the Daily Value is 5% or less, the food only adds a small amount of that nutrient. But, if the Daily Value is above 20%, the food gives you quite a bit of that nutrient. For example, a frozen dinner gives you 13% of your fat grams for the day. If you use the rule above, 13% is a moderate amount. Consider the food and how you will use it. Is it a main course, like this frozen dinner, or is it a snack? If 1 serving of a snack, such as microwave popcorn, has 13% of your fat for the day, that is pretty high. You might want to find a lower-fat version of your snack or have a lower-fat dinner to balance the fat that you ate in the snack.

Nutrition claims tell all

You can believe what you read on the Nutrition Fact panel. However, don't be taken in by the big bold print on the front of the package. When a manufacturer makes a nutrition claim, the information supporting the claim must be in the Nutrition Facts panel.

For the health of it

Only a few health claims can be used, and only those for which there is scientific evidence. A health claim describes the relationship between a food or nutrient and a disease, such as fat and cancer. Currently, no health claims are directly related to diabetes.

To buy or not to buy

Before you drop a new food in your shopping cart, read the label carefully, and answer these questions:

▲ Is the portion realistic for you, or will you need to count it as more than 1 serving?

▲ How many calories are in a serving?

▲ How many grams of fat are in a serving? What is your daily value for fat?

▲ Does the advertising on the front match the Nutrition Facts?

▲ Does the food fit into your meal plan and, if so, in what food group or groups?

▲ Are you comfortable with this food in the house, or is it better to avoid the temptation?

▲ If it is a convenience, ready-to-eat food that is likely to be expensive, can you make it at home? A homemade recipe can be less expensive, be lower in calories and sodium, and have fewer additives. Examples are low-calorie hot cocoa mix, popcorn, soup, and pasta dishes.

Guides for the aisles

Here are some purchasing guidelines to help you read labels and do comparison shopping for the best nutrition:

▲ Grains

Buy your favorites and try new ones.

They are dry and store easily and for a long time.

They have little or no fat and are easy to prepare.

▲ Hot cereals

Have a few on hand.

Add skim milk in cooking and when eating for more calcium.

▲ Dry cereal

Look for 4–5 g dietary fiber per serving.

Keep the sugars under 5–6 g per serving and fat below 1–2 g.

Keep a stash of individual boxes to use as quick meals or snacks on the run.

▲ Pasta, noodles

Buy the dry—they are least expensive and store the longest.

Purchase the whole-wheat or whole-grain variety for extra fiber.

▲ Breads, bagels, rolls, etc.

Go for whole wheat or whole-grain varieties. Get at least 2–3 g dietary fiber per serving.

Cut the fat by limiting biscuits, croissants, and doughnuts.

▲ Crackers

Buy fat-free and reduced-fat types, but be sure they really are.

Keep fat to 1–2 g per serving.

Buy whole grain to get 1–2 g dietary fiber per serving.

▲ Starchy snack foods

Go for the naturally fat free—pretzels and baked tortilla chips.

Purchase light, fat-free, and reduced-fat varieties, but make sure they are what they say.

▲ Beans

Have several types of dried beans on hand. They store well.

Stock a few types of canned beans.

They have zero fat and plenty of soluble fiber.

Buy fat-free varieties of refried beans, baked beans, and vegetarian chili.

▲ Starchy vegetables

Have potatoes on hand to cook in the microwave—whole or chopped.

Try red (new) potatoes or Yukon gold for a small, sweet, tasty variety.

Buy fresh sweet potatoes and squashes; they stay fresh for several weeks and are packed with vitamins and minerals.

Keep canned or frozen corn and peas.

▲ Vegetables

Eat fresh often.

Keep canned or frozen ones so you'll always have vegetables.

Avoid high-fat sauces and seasonings on frozen vegetables.

Keep individual cans of vegetable juice on hand for a quick dose of vegetables.

▲ Fruits

Eat fresh, whole pieces of fruit often.

Keep canned or frozen so you'll always have fruit.

Buy no-sugar-added, packed-in-its-own-juice, canned, or frozen fruit.

If you buy fruit juice, look for 100% fruit juice.

Avoid fruit drinks and fruit-flavored carbonated drinks with a lot of calories.

▲ Milk and yogurt

Your watch words are *skim*, *nonfat*, and *fat free*.

For yogurt, choose nonfat, sugar free; fat free, sugar free; or nonfat (higher sugars content).

▲ Red meats—beef, lamb, pork, and veal

Choose the leaner cuts as often as possible.

Go for lean or extra-lean ground meat.

Buy lean or extra-lean cold cuts, hot dogs.

▲ Poultry

The skinless breast with no wing is lowest in fat.

Try turkey parts.

Buy ground turkey or low-fat turkey sausage to replace ground meat in recipes. Check the label; ground turkey with the skin included is higher in fat.

Usually a whole bird is cheapest, and boneless breast is most expensive per pound.

▲ Seafood

Keep canned tuna (water packed), salmon, crabmeat, or imitation crabmeat on hand for a quick meal.

Buy any type of fresh or frozen unbreaded.

▲ Cheese

Go for cheeses with less than 5 g fat per oz—*part skim* and *reduced calorie* are the watch words.

Cottage cheese—buy 1%, nonfat, or fat-free.

▲ Fats

Oil—keep olive and canola oil for monounsaturated fat.

Margarine/spreads—a light, tub variety (about 5 g fat per Tbsp). Or make your own by whipping 1 cup of butter and 1 cup of mild tasting oil together.

Mayonnaise—low fat or reduced calorie (about 5 g fat per Tbsp).

Salad dressing—reduced calorie (about 5 g fat per 2 Tbsp) or fat free (less than 20–30 calories per 2 Tbsp).

Sour cream, cream cheese—light or fat-free types.

▲ Cookies, cakes

Only keep ones that you can control the portions you eat.

Try fat-free desserts, but remember they are not calorie free!

▲ Frozen desserts

Buy light and fat-free varieties, but remember they are not calorie free.

Keep calories in the 100–150 range per 1/2-cup serving.

▲ Free foods

Keep plenty of fat-free items in the pantry.

These add flavor to low-fat meals.

▲ Soups

Keep cans or dry packages for quick meals or snacks.

Limit creamy varieties.

Dry packages work well as a traveling meal or snack.

Dry packages of vegetable, onion, or others can double as dip mix. (Watch sodium content.)

▲ Frozen entrees

Buy reduced-calorie varieties to limit fat and keep serving sizes under control.

Keep fat down to about 3 g per 100 g of food.

Keep sodium down to 600–800 mg per entree.

▲ Pizza

Keep a frozen cheese variety on hand, and top with vegetables. Purchase a pizza crust, pita bread, or bagel, and add your own tomato sauce, part-skim cheese, and vegetables.

Now you know

▲ What you can find on the food label.

▲ What you can find on the Nutrition Facts panel.

▲ How to use the information you find on the label to make healthy food choices.

▲ Some guidelines to follow when you are in the supermarket.

Scenario

Meet Patricia. She has had type II diabetes for about 2 years and was diagnosed when she was 52 years old. She has been struggling to lose the 15–20 pounds her doctor says will help her control her blood glucose and blood fats. Her goal is 165 pounds, and she is 5'7". She also has problems with regularity.

Her doctor suggested that foods with lots of dietary fiber would help her constipation and maybe lower her blood fats a bit. Patricia had not met with a dietitian until some members of a diabetes support group said that a few visits with a dietitian had helped them. Patricia made an appointment.

They talked about Patricia's weight loss, blood glucose records, blood fats, and problems with constipation. The dietitian asked Patricia about the foods she buys in the supermarket and whether she understands and uses nutrition information.

They found that Patricia was not eating certain foods because she was applying the 30% fat rule to every food. They figured Patricia's daily value for fat is 60 g based on about 1800 calories each day. They looked at a few food labels, and Patricia learned how to add up the total grams of fat. She also learned to compute the calories from fat and how that adds to her total calories. She now realizes that she can enjoy reduced-calorie salad dressing, mayonnaise, and light sour cream in the proper servings as long as her total fat intake is around 50–60 g per day or 25–30% of her total calories.

Patricia and the dietitian also looked at how she could increase dietary fiber to help ease constipation and lower blood fats. They determined her daily value for dietary fiber is 21 g. The dietitian suggested Patricia try to sprinkle peas, garbanzo beans, kidney beans, or bulgur wheat on salads; buy dry cereals that have at least 5–6 g of fiber; and buy whole-grain breads with a few grams of dietary fiber. She also suggested trying for at least 5 servings of fruits and vegetables each day. Patricia agreed to chart her progress and come back in 1 month.

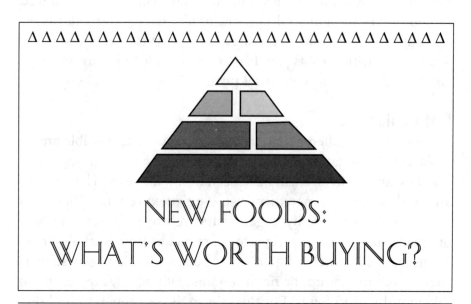

CHAPTER 17

NEW FOODS:
WHAT'S WORTH BUYING?

What you will learn

▲ What are the new healthy foods and the words that help you spot them.

▲ Why it is hard to manufacture these foods.

▲ What are fat replacers.

▲ What are low-calorie sweeteners (sugar substitutes).

▲ What's in the crystal ball for new food ingredients.

▲ Fat free does not mean calorie free.

▲ Sugar free does not mean calorie free.

What are the new healthy foods?

It seems like you see more new "healthy" products on each trip to the supermarket, with sugar-free, reduced-calorie, and low-fat advertising on the label. No longer can you simply decide on the flavor of salad dressing you want. First you have to choose among regular, reduced calorie, or fat free.

Just a few years ago, only a few so-called dietetic or diabetic foods were available, and they were all in a small section of one supermarket aisle. The new foods we're talking about are foods that have been changed to be in line with today's nutrition recommendations. Many are reduced in fat or fat free, some are reduced in cholesterol or saturated fat, and others have fewer calories or less sugars. These foods can show up anywhere on the shelves. Read the Nutrition Facts panel and ingredient list to know whether and how they fit into your meal plan.

Fat replacers

Many of the ingredients that make these new foods possible are fat replacers. Most fat replacers in foods are made from sugars or starches, and many of them have been in use for years. Their names are on thousands of ingredient lists—polydextrose, modified food starch, maltodextrins, hydrogenated starch hydrolysate, xanthan, or guar gum. These fat replacers are made from carbohydrate. Sometimes it is starch, often corn or potato; simple sugars such as sucrose or corn syrup; or natural gums. Different fat replacers do different things in foods. For this reason, it is common to find several in one food. Here is an example of the ingredient list from a fat-free salad dressing with the carbohydrate-based fat replacers noted in bold:

Fat-free French salad dressing:

Water, sugar, tomato paste, vinegar, soybean oil, salt, **hydrolyzed rice, food starch–modified**, honey, lemon juice, whey protein concentrate, **xanthan gum**, garlic powder, flavoring.

Fat replacers and diabetes

When you have diabetes, you must ask what these carbohydrate-based fat replacers do to your blood glucose levels. If you substitute fat-free cream cheese that has no fat and some carbohydrate for regular cream cheese that has fat and very little carbohydrate, what is the impact on your blood glucose?

Because carbohydrate raises blood glucose quicker and higher than fat, you might see a difference when you measure your blood glucose. Discuss the foods you eat with your dietitian. He or she can help you work these foods into your meal plan.

Fat replacers of the future

Simplesse, a protein-based fat replacer, was approved by the FDA in 1990 and is used in a few reduced-calorie and reduced-fat cheeses and several other foods. In the future, there will probably be more protein-based fat replacers like Simplesse. However, the greatest growth will be in the development of fat-based fat replacers. Many companies are at work on these, but only one company, Procter and Gamble, has received approval for their fat-based fat replacer olestra, or Olean, as it is called on ingredients lists.

Simple Facts about Olestra

Olestra is made from sugar and fat. It acts like any other fat in cooking or baking. But once olestra gets into the body, it works differently from regular fat. Fats in foods have just 3 (tri) fatty acids. Olestra has 6–8 fatty acids. These extra fatty acids make it impossible for the enzymes that usually break up fat molecules to break up olestra. So, olestra goes through the intestine undigested, and the body does not get the calories from the fat. What could be better—fat without the calories?

Because some scientists have voiced concerns about olestra's effect on the body, the FDA requires that vitamins be added and that this label be put on all foods containing olestra:

> This product contains olestra. Olestra may cause abdominal cramping and loose stools [diarrhea]. Olestra inhibits the absorption of some vitamins and other nutrients. Vitamins A, D, E, and K have been added.

In 1998, FDA will review olestra's effects on consumers. It's up to you to see whether your body handles it okay. It is important to remember that these foods still contain calories from other ingredients.

None of the sugars

Sugars make foods sweet. Sugars also play a role in the structure and texture of foods; lower the freezing point, which is important for frozen desserts; and help to keep foods moist and tender.

Sugar substitutes, or low-calorie sweeteners, have been around for years. In fact, saccharin dates back to the late 1800s. Low-calorie sweeteners don't have the calories of sugar, yet give the food the sweetness of sugar. Today, three low-calorie sweeteners are used in the United States—acesulfame-k (Sunette), aspartame (NutraSweet), and saccharin. Aspartame, because of its sugar-like taste, continues to be used in the greatest number of sugar-free and reduced-sugar foods, such as diet soda, tabletop packets, sugar-free hot cocoa mix, regular and frozen yogurt, and ice cream. The main use of saccharin these days is in fountain diet soda (coupled with aspartame) and in tabletop packets. Acesulfame-k is in a few products like sugarless gum and iced tea mix. It is used more internationally, where it is often blended with aspartame or saccharin.

What about sugar alcohols

Other foods that can be called sugar free on the food label are sweetened with sugar alcohols. Sugar alcohols, also called polyols, are sorbitol, mannitol, and xylitol. They are used in the candies and cookies often found in the diabetic foods section of the supermarket. You also see sorbitol used as a "bulking ingredient" in fat-free, sugar-free foods. Are they better for you? The nutrition recommendations say that sugar alcohols are no better than other calorie-containing sweeteners, such as sugar. Plus sugar alcohols can cause stomach problems like cramps and diarrhea if you eat large amounts. Do not think that foods with sugar alcohols are calorie free or carbohydrate free.

Not a calorie-free ride

Foods with fat replacers, low-calorie sweeteners, or sugar alcohols have calories. Those calories are from the carbohydrate of the fat replacer as well as from other ingredients in the food.

Consider the nutrition label from a sugar- and fat-free hot cocoa mix:

> ## Hot Cocoa Mix
> ## Nutrition Facts
>
> Serving size   1 envelope, 6–8 oz
>
> **Servings per container   1**
>
> ---
>
> **Calories 25**
>
> **Total fat   0g**
>
> **Cholesterol   79mg**
>
> **Sodium   135mg**
>
> **Total carbohydrate   4g**
>
>   Dietary fiber   1g
>
>   Sugars   3g (from lactose)
>
> **Protein   2g**

So, if in an average day you use several servings of fat-free or sugar-free foods, the calories can add up.

A few helpful guidelines

Now you know that many fat-free and sugar-free foods have calories. Here are helpful guidelines from the American Diabetes Association for counting these foods in your meal plan. These guidelines are especially important if weight loss is one of your diabetes goals.

▲ A food or drink with fat replacers or low-calorie sweeteners that has 20 calories or less or 5 g of carbohydrate or less in each serving is not likely to raise your blood glucose or add significant calories. These foods are free foods.

▲ Limit the use of sugar-free or fat-free foods (free foods) with more than 20 calories or 5 g of carbohydrate to 3 servings each day. Spread these servings out over the day.

▲ If a sugar-free or fat-free food has more than 20 calories and more than 5 g of carbohydrate per serving, count it as part of your meal plan.

▲ If the calories are mainly from carbohydrate, count them as follows:

6–10 g of carbohydrate as 1/2 starch, fruit, or milk serving (whichever fits the food).

11–20 g of carbohydrate as 1 starch, fruit, or milk serving (whichever fits the food).

▲ If the calories are from fat, carbohydrate, or protein, use the directions on page 125 to figure out how to fit the food into your meal plan.

Examples:

How to count frozen yogurt:

   1/2 cup = 23 g carbohydrate = 1 serving starch

Frozen Yogurt: fat-free
Nutrition Facts
Serving size 1/2 cup or 4 oz
Calories 110
Total fat   0g
Sodium   105mg
Total carbohydrate   23g
Dietary fiber   1g
Sugars   13g (from lactose)
Protein   4g

A food that contains carbohydrate will fit into the grains, beans, and starchy vegetables; or milk; or fruit section on the pyramid. Divide the amount of carbohydrate in the food by the 15 g carbohydrate in 1 pyramid serving. Divide 15 into 23 to see how many pyramid servings are in your serving of yogurt.

   23/15 = 1 1/2 servings from grains, beans, and starchy vegetables, or milk and yogurt.

How to count fat-free mayonnaise:

   1 Tbsp = free   2 Tbsp = 8 g carbohydrate

Mayonnaise

Nutrition Facts

Serving size 1 Tbsp

Calories 25	
Total fat 1g	
Sodium 140mg	
Total carbohydrate 4g	
Sugars 3g	
Protein 0g	

A food that contains carbohydrate will fit into the grains, beans, and starchy vegetables; or the milk; or the fruit section on the pyramid. Divide the amount of carbohydrate in the food by the 15 g carbohydrate in 1 pyramid serving.

8/15 = 1/2 serving of grains, beans, and starchy vegetables; or milk; or fruit.

New foods—helpful or harmful

New foods can help you eat more fruits, vegetables, and starches by adding a variety of tastes. Think of fat-free, sugar-free fruited yogurt on fresh strawberries or fat-free sour cream with fresh herbs on a baked potato or steamed broccoli.

Some of these foods can satisfy your sweet tooth without adding many calories—hot cocoa, frozen yogurt, or a popsicle. But, you must remember that fat free or sugar free does not mean calorie free. Read the nutrition facts and only have one serving.

Now you know

▲ The definition of new foods.
▲ Which fat replacers are used today and their impact on blood glucose.
▲ Which low-calorie sweeteners are used today.
▲ Which fat replacers and low-calorie sweeteners to look for in the future.
▲ Sugar free does not mean calorie free.
▲ Fat free does not mean calorie free.

Scenario

Meet Joseph. He has had type II diabetes for a year. It was diagnosed 2 weeks after his youngest daughter was married. Joseph is 5'9" and 210 pounds—50 pounds overweight. He is 69, is retired, and lives by himself. His doctor pleads with him to lose 10 or 20 pounds, saying it will improve his blood glucose, cholesterol, and blood pressure.

Joseph complains of joint pain in his hips and knees. His doctor says that losing weight will ease his pain. Joseph has been trying to cut down on fats and sweets, but he only lost 5–6 pounds last year. His doctor encouraged him to see an RD.

When Joseph told the RD what he ate day to day, he mentioned how he is careful to buy fat-free cookies, salad dressing, and mayonnaise and sugar-free hard candies and hot cocoa mix. The RD asked if he looked at the calories in these foods. Joseph said he pays more attention to the total fats and sugars on the Nutrition Facts panel. The RD agreed that it is important to count fat and sugar, but it is just as important to eat only a certain number of calories each day to lose weight. They added up the calories from his healthy food choices in a day:

Food	Calories
2 tsp sugar-free jam	16
1 serving fat-free salad dressing	30
1 envelope hot cocoa mix	25
2 Tbsp fat-free cream cheese	25
1 Tbsp fat-free mayonnaise	13
2 fat-free cookies	100
2 sugar-free hard candies	20
Total	230

Joseph was amazed at the 230 extra calories from foods he thought were calorie free. He was getting a lot of extra calories from these so-called freebies. The dietitian encouraged Joseph to focus on serving sizes, calories, total fat, and sugars. He suggested some questions for Joseph to ask himself before buying the food.

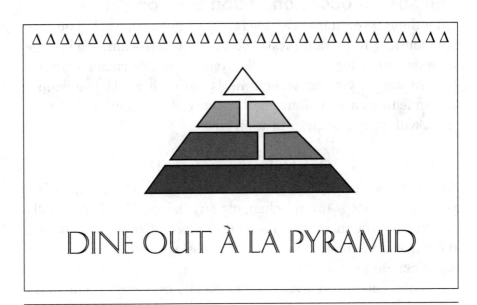

CHAPTER 18

DINE OUT À LA PYRAMID

What you will learn

▲ How much, when, what, and why YOU eat out.

▲ Reasons it can be difficult to eat healthfully in a restaurant.

▲ Strategies to help you eat healthfully away from home.

▲ How to use the food pyramid to plan restaurant menus.

▲ Healthier choices in a variety of restaurants.

Restaurant eating—an American pastime

Twenty years ago a restaurant meal was reserved for a special occasion—Mother's Day, a birthday, an anniversary. Today, restaurant meals can happen every day. Maybe you pick up a quick bagel, banana, and coffee in the morning and stop by the rotisserie-chicken store on your way home from work. A lunch out with fellow workers makes you three for three.

Restaurant eating is a way of life. On average, Americans eat four meals out each week. It is no surprise that about one-quarter of these meals are fast foods. We eat out for many reasons—not enough time to prepare food at home, no food in the house, the desire to eat a particular type of food, or the desire to relax after a long day. So, it is time to master the art of dining out à la pyramid.

The special occasion notion lives on

Even though you might eat several meals out each week, you may still consider restaurant meals special occasions—times to splurge on a dessert, a high-fat extra like french fries, or cream sauce on the chicken. If you eat several meals out each week, you cannot continue to view restaurant meals as special occasions and stay on track with your diabetes nutrition goals.

Get to know yourself

As we've said before, you need to learn what you're doing before you can take steps toward changing any habits. That is especially true for restaurant eating. Take out a piece of paper and answer these questions about your restaurant eating habits:

▲ **When** do I eat out?

–Think about an average day, week, or month (whichever applies to you); estimate the number of meals and snacks you eat away from home. Do not forget meals and snacks that you purchase at restaurants and eat somewhere else.

–Compare how often you eat out on weekdays and weekends.

▲ **What** meals and snacks do I eat away from home during an average day, week, or month (whichever applies to you)?

–Breakfast, lunch, dinner

–Morning, afternoon, evening/bedtime snack

▲ **Why** do I eat restaurant meals?

–Restaurant meals are convenient.

–No time, and restaurant meals are quick.

–Do not like to cook.

–Want to have someone serve me.

–Enjoy various ethnic flavors that I cannot create in my kitchen.

–Need a place and way to get together with friends, family, or business associates.

–Want to relax during lunch or at dinner after a long day.

▲ **What** types of restaurants do I choose?

–Fast food (hamburger, chicken, or seafood chains)

–Pizza/sub shops

—American fare—family restaurant, steak house, upscale continental cuisine
—Ethnic fare (fast food)
—Ethnic fare (table service)
—Sweets/desserts/ice cream

▲ **What** foods do I eat in the restaurants listed above and in what amounts?
   —Write down what you usually order in the restaurants you go to (including beverages).

▲ **Observe** the foods you eat at different types of restaurants.
   —How do the servings compare with the servings on my pyramid meal plan?
   —Are there food groups missing from restaurant meals that should be part of my meal plan?

▲ **Do** I drink alcoholic beverages when I eat in restaurants?
   —If yes, how many alcoholic drinks do I have when I eat out?
   —What alcoholic beverages do I usually drink?
   —What is the calorie content of these alcoholic beverages?

Change...one step at a time

Use the information you gathered from the above questions to take steps toward healthier restaurant eating. If you found out that you drive through a fast-food restaurant to pick up a high-fat sausage biscuit more often than you would like to admit, then set some concrete goals to change that habit.

If you see that you are caught in the cycle of eating out often because you do not keep healthy foods at home, then attack that problem. If you see that your usual order has high fat and calories and the servings are large, then think how to make that menu selection healthier. You might find that you need to save a few of your favorite restaurants for a once-a-year splurge.

Challenges to eating healthfully in restaurants

There are three main challenges to eating healthy in restaurants. The first challenge is the high-fat and high-calorie content of restaurant foods. By now you know that fat makes food taste good.

Restaurants love to use oils or shortening to fry; butter and cream to create sauces; salad dressing on salad; sour cream on baked potatoes; cheese or cheese sauce on sandwiches; and butter, cream, and eggs to make desserts. You'll need the strategies below.

Please note that restaurant foods can be high in sodium as well as fat and calories. The high sodium content comes from salt, ingredients like soy sauce, meat tenderizers, broth, ham or bacon; sauces and gravies; use of prepared canned food such as soups and vegetables; and salad dressings. If you need to limit sodium, you may have to eat out less often. When you do eat out, limit high-sodium foods just as you do in the supermarket. Asian cuisines—Japanese, Chinese, and Thai—are all high in sodium.

Challenge number two is the large serving of protein (meat, poultry, or seafood) you usually get. This is particularly hard to avoid in American-style restaurants—steak houses, delicatessens, sandwich shops, and family restaurants. How about a delicatessen sandwich stuffed with 6–8 oz of corned beef, pastrami, or smoked turkey? You know from the food pyramid that is enough meat for two or three sandwiches. To eat healthfully in restaurants, you need to "outsmart" the menu to have a reasonable serving of meat. You will learn techniques to do this below.

Challenge number three is larger servings than anyone needs to eat. Generally, meals in restaurants are about double the food that most adults need. Unfortunately, in America, we think that more food equals greater value. It is economically wise to buy the "value" meal or to go to the all-you-can-eat buffet, but it's not nutritionally wise.

Strategies to eat healthier in restaurants

▲ Have a can-do attitude: If you believe that a restaurant meal is a special occasion, but you eat out four to seven times a week, then you need to admit it. It's OK. You do have the ability to eat a healthy restaurant meal and please your taste buds at the same time.

▲ Select a restaurant with care: Today, you can go into most restaurants and choose to eat healthfully. The accent is on the words *you* and *choose*. Either the menu lists healthier items or you can design a healthy meal by being creative with the menu. It is your choice. Granted, there are restaurants where every food is fried. Do not set yourself up for defeat, select restaurants that offer you at least a few healthy options.

▲ Have a game plan: When you cross the threshold of a restaurant have in mind what you will order.

▲ Be a knowledgeable fat detective: You know that restaurant foods load on the fat. It is easy to keep a lid on fats if you learn:
  –The foods that are high in fats and calories, such as
    butter, cream, mayonnaise, sour cream, salad dressing, cheese, sausage, nuts, and avocado.
  –The cooking methods described on the menu that add
    fat, such as, fried, deep-fried, battered and fried, golden brown, sautéed in butter, and served in a cream sauce.
  –The names of high-fat dishes, such as chimichangas
    (Mexican), fettuccini Alfredo (Italian), and sweet and sour (Chinese).

▲ Hold the line on fats: Once you can spot the high-fat offenders, steer clear or cut down on them.

Now for the terms that mean healthy:

▲ Menu descriptions, such as broth-based tomato sauce, with lettuce and tomato, fat-free or low-calorie salad dressing, fresh fruit. Some foods are naturally low in fat and calories, such as, vegetables, pasta, dried beans, herbs, and spices.

▲ The cooking methods and menu descriptions, such as marinated, poached, grilled, blackened, served in a light wine sauce, and topped with sautéed garden vegetables.

▲ The names of dishes such as fajitas (Mexican dish with guacamole and sour cream that you can request held or on the side), Yu Hsiang chicken (Chinese), and pasta primavera (be careful the sauce does not have cream added).

▲ Be creative with the menu: Do not feel that you have to order an entree if the portions seem huge. If restaurants want to serve too much food, then order from the appetizer, soup, salad, and side dishes.

▲ Split menu items: Because servings are so large, there is often enough for two. (You might need to order an extra side dish.) For example, one person orders an 8-oz (raw weight) sirloin steak, a baked potato, and a trip to the salad bar. The other person orders an extra baked potato and trip to the salad bar. Split the steak. That is just the right size, about 3 oz cooked meat for each person.

▲ Good news for "splitters" is that in many ethnic restaurants, family-style service is customary. That means that the entire dish is placed in the middle of the table to share. You decide how large your serving will be. Order one or two fewer dishes than the number of people dining.

▲ You can split with yourself as well. Order a menu item with a doggie bag. When your order arrives, put half away to take home or to the office for another meal.

▲ Share menu items: Share two or more menu items (depending on the number of dining partners) that complement each other and achieve the goals of your food pyramid meal plan. This technique outsmarts the large protein servings. For example, in an Italian restaurant, one dining partner orders chicken cacciatore, which will probably have about 6–8 oz of chicken, or 3–4 oz when you split the dish. The other partner orders pasta with a light tomato sauce, marinara or bolognese. Split this dish so each of you ends up with 1–1 1/2 cups of pasta. Order your own dinner salad for more vegetables.

▲ Order foods as you want them: Special requests help you trim the fat and calories. It's OK to make reasonable requests, but don't ask that a menu item be re-created. For example, do not request that a fried dish like Chicken Kiev be grilled. Move on to a healthier item such as grilled teriyaki chicken or stir-fry chicken with garden vegetables served over linguine. Here are some reasonable special requests:

    –Please bring my salad dressing, butter, or sour cream on the side.

    –Please remove from the table, or do not bring, any bread and butter, chips and salsa, or Chinese noodles.

–Can the chef grill or broil this meat (poultry or seafood) rather than fry it?

–Please hold the sour cream, guacamole, shredded cheese, or olives.

–Please split this entree into 2 servings in the kitchen, or bring us an extra plate.

–Can you serve this ham or turkey sandwich on whole wheat bread rather than a croissant?

–Can you hold the mayonnaise and bring me mustard?

Let the pyramid be your guide

Picture some restaurant meals. A fast-food quarter-pound hamburger, french fries, side salad with thousand island dressing, and a regular soda. Or a Mexican meal with a basket of chips and salsa, then a combo plate with one chicken taco, one beef enchilada, Mexican rice, refried beans, and a dessert of custard flan. Both these meals turn the pyramid upside down. They are heavy on fats, meats, and sweets and light on milk, vegetables, and starches. Fruits are nowhere to be seen.

Let the food pyramid and your own meal plan help you. You want to go heavy on the starches, vegetables, fruits, and milk and light on the meats, fats, and sweets. Apply the strategies of healthy restaurant eating, be creative with the menu, and make special requests to get foods as you want them.

With a menu in hand, keep a mental picture of the food pyramid. Order to mesh with your meal plan for that meal or snack. You could make a little copy of your meal plan with the number of servings from each food group that you need for each meal and snack. Keep this in your wallet as a handy reference when you eat away from home.

The following examples show you how to match the number of servings from meal plans based on the food pyramid with sample meals from a variety of restaurants:

Fast-food lunch based on 1200 calories a day

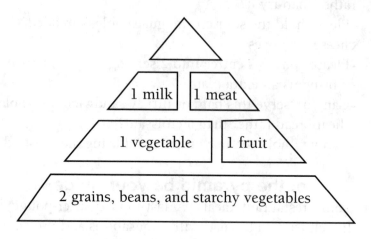

Hamburger (small)   2 starches
                                           1 meat
Garden salad   1 vegetable
  with light vinaigrette (2 Tbsp)   free food
Low-fat or skim milk
  (1/2 pint, 8 oz)   1 milk
1 small apple (bring from home)   1 fruit

Nutrition Facts	
Calories 502	
Total fat 13g	
Cholesterol 47mg	
Sodium 1072mg	
Total carbohydrate 57g	
Protein 29g	

Dinner at an Italian restaurant based on about 1400 calories a day

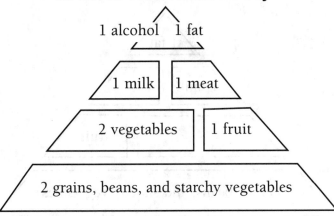

1 alcohol   1 fat

1 milk   1 meat

2 vegetables   1 fruit

2 grains, beans, and starchy vegetables

Shrimp cocktail (3 oz)	1 meat
with cocktail sauce (2 Tbsp)	free food
Pasta (1 cup)	2 starches
with light tomato sauce	1 vegetable
Garden salad	1 vegetable
with oil (1 tsp)	5 g fat
and vinegar	free food
Strawberries and	1 fruit
1 oz berry liqueur	1 alcohol

Nutrition Facts

Calories 660	
Total fat 15g	
Cholesterol 181mg	
Sodium 1221mg	
Total carbohydrate 88g	
Protein 32g	

Breakfast at a coffee shop based on about 1600 calories a day

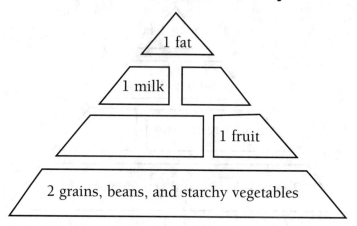

1 fat

1 milk

1 fruit

2 grains, beans, and starchy vegetables

Bagel (small/2.5 oz)   2 starches
  [**Note:** Many bagels purchased
  in shops are 3–4 oz]
 with light, reduced-fat
   cream cheese (2 Tbsp)   5 g fat
Banana (small/4 oz)   1 fruit
Yogurt, nonfat (3/4 cup)   1 milk

Nutrition Facts	
Calories 410	
Total fat 6g	
Cholesterol 14mg	
Sodium 668mg	
Total carbohydrate 69g	
Protein 21g	

Dinner at pizza parlor based on about 1800 calories a day

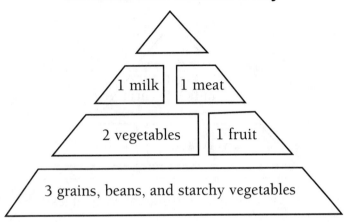

2 slices cheese pizza   3 starches
   with vegetables,   1 vegetable
   thin crust   1 meat
1 garden salad   1 vegetable
   with low-calorie Italian dressing   free food
      (2 Tbsp)
Frozen yogurt, soft serve (1/3 cup)   sweet (milk)
   with fresh fruit topping (1/2 cup)   1 fruit

Nutrition Facts

Calories	690
Total fat	24g
Cholesterol	53mg
Sodium	1515mg
Total carbohydrate	81g
Protein	35g

Lunch at rotisserie-chicken chain store based on about 2200 calories a day

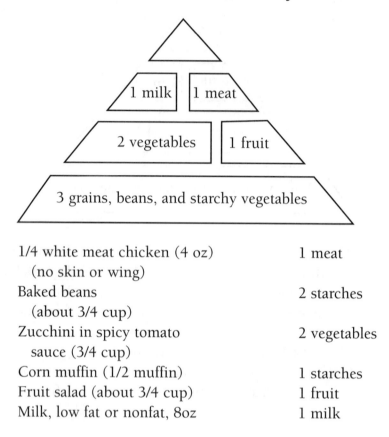

1/4 white meat chicken (4 oz) (no skin or wing)	1 meat
Baked beans (about 3/4 cup)	2 starches
Zucchini in spicy tomato sauce (3/4 cup)	2 vegetables
Corn muffin (1/2 muffin)	1 starches
Fruit salad (about 3/4 cup)	1 fruit
Milk, low fat or nonfat, 8oz	1 milk

Note: several servings are larger than the servings suggested in the food pyramid, as is usual with restaurant-size servings.

Nutrition Facts
Calories 700
Total fat 19g
Cholesterol 119mg
Sodium 1557mg
Total carbohydrate 92g
Protein 52g

Dinner at Mexican restaurant based on about 2800 calories a day

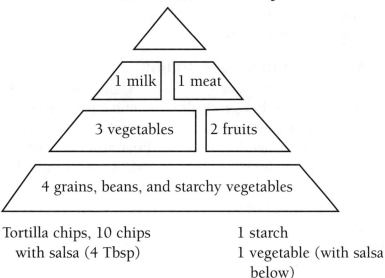

Tortilla chips, 10 chips   1 starch
  with salsa (4 Tbsp)   1 vegetable (with salsa below)

Chicken soft taco, no sour   1 starch
  cream or guacamole   1/2 meat
  add lettuce, tomato, and onions   1 vegetable
Bean burrito   3 starches*
  add vegetables   1 vegetable
  extra salsa on side (6 Tbsp)   1 vegetable (with salsa above)

Milk, low fat or nonfat, 8 oz   1 milk

*One starch (15 g carbohydrate) substitutes for 1 fruit (15 g carbohydrate) serving. Eat the other fruit serving soon after this meal.

Nutrition Facts	
Calories 996	
Total fat 32g	
Cholesterol 72mg	
Sodium 2520mg	
Total carbohydrate 139g	
Protein 46g	

Healthier choices in restaurants

In this list, healthier selections follow the food pyramid—heavy on starches and vegetables and light on meats. Unhealthy selections are high in meat and fats.

Fast-food hamburger chains

Healthier choices	Unhealthy choices
Hamburger, cheeseburger, single	Hamburger, cheeseburger, double, triple, deluxe
Grilled chicken sandwich	
Grilled chicken salad	Fried fish sandwich
Baked potato, with chili or broccoli	Baked potato with cheese sauce
French fries, small or share	
Garden and side salads	
Chef salad (light dressing)	
Roast beef sandwich	
Frozen yogurt	

Rotisserie-chicken chains

Healthier choices	Unhealthy choices
White meat, rotisserie, BBQ, grilled	Dark meat, with skin
Ham or Turkey	Chicken, fried
Chicken soup	Chicken pie
Side dishes	Side dishes
apples and cinnamon	Caesar salad with dressing
corn bread or muffin	coleslaw
baked beans	creamed spinach
corn	macaroni and cheese
fruit salad	pasta salad
green beans	stuffing
potatoes, mashed, pieces, baked	
rice	Meat sandwiches with cheese sauce
steamed vegetables	
zucchini in tomato sauce	Chicken salad sandwiches

Mexican

Healthier choices	Unhealthy choices
Black bean, tortilla soup, or gazpacho	Chili con queso
Mexican or taco salad	Chimichangas
Arroz con pollo (chicken and rice)	Flautas
Burritos	Nachos or super nachos
Enchiladas	Tacos (hard shell)
Fajitas	
Soft tacos	

Side dishes:
  Black beans
  Mexican rice
  Pico de gallo

> Note: To eat less fat, ask for cheese, sour cream, or guacamole on the side. Request extra salsa to add flavor.

Chinese

Healthier choices	Unhealthy choices
Wonton, egg drop, or hot and sour soup	Egg or spring roll
Steamed Peking dumpling	Spareribs
Teriyaki beef or chicken	Jumbo shrimp
Chop suey or chow mein	Meat and nut dishes
Moo shi chicken, etc.	Deep-fried dishes
Shrimp with tomato sauce	General Tso's chicken
Vegetarian stir-fry dishes	Sweet and sour shrimp, chicken, etc.
	Peking duck

Italian

Healthier choices	Unhealthy choices
Italian bread (hold the butter)	Garlic bread
Marinated vegetable salad	Fried mozzarella cheese sticks
Minestrone soup	Caesar salad with dressing
Shrimp cocktail	Canneloni, lasagna
Pasta with tomato sauce, marinara, bolognese, meatballs, red or white clam sauce	Pasta with pesto
	Sausage and peppers

Italian

Healthier choices

Chicken or veal with cacciatore, light wine, or light tomato sauce

Chicken or shrimp primavera (no cream in the sauce)

Unhealthy choices

Pasta with cream and cheese sauces, Alfredo, carbonara

Chicken or veal parmigiana

Pizza and Submarine Shop

Healthier choices

Cheese pizza with vegetables

Submarine sandwiches with turkey, ham, roast beef, cheese (hold the oil and mayonnaise, and add vegetables)

Unhealthy choices

Cheese pizza with sausage, pepperoni, and/or extra cheese

Submarine sandwiches with tuna, chicken, or seafood salad; Italian cold cuts

American restaurants

Healthier choices

Broth-based soup

Chili

Peel and eat shrimp

Salad with light or fat-free salad dressing (on the side)

Salad with grilled tuna or chicken

Baked potato topped with chili

Fajitas

Stir-fry chicken with vegetables

Teriyaki chicken breast

Unhealthy choices

New England clam chowder

French onion soup

Buffalo wings

Potato skins

Tuna melt

Philadelphia cheese steak

Quiche

Ribs—beef or pork

Now you know

▲ How much, when, what, and why YOU eat out.

▲ Restaurant meals are generally high in fat, the portions are large and full of protein (meat, poultry, or seafood).

▲ The strategies to eat healthier when you eat out.

▲ How to order restaurant meals à la pyramid.

▲ Healthier choices in a variety of restaurants.

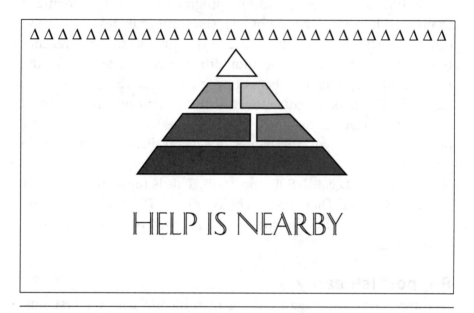

CHAPTER 19

HELP IS NEARBY

Shape your pyramid

Choose healthy foods that are tasty and enjoyable. Eating should be fun. Try the easy ways suggested in this book to eat more starches, fruits, and vegetables, and explore the tips to trim unwanted fat. You're on your way to an adventure in good eating and shaping your personal pyramid.

There is always something new to learn about diabetes. Meal planning and blood glucose testing are two actions that will help you live healthier every day with diabetes.

Remember that new lifestyle changes come slowly but surely as long as you take a can-do attitude. Tackle easy habits first, and reward yourself for your successes. You'll have many.

Where to find help

The three 800 numbers listed on the next page can help you find a diabetes education program and diabetes educators. In addition, ask your doctor to refer you to a diabetes educator, or call a local hospital and ask about diabetes educators or a diabetes education program. Attend a local diabetes support group, and ask people there to recommend a diabetes educator or education program.

To find a diabetes education program that is a Recognized Diabetes Education program by the American Diabetes Association call 1-800-DIA-BETES (800-342-2383). This toll-free call reaches the American Diabetes Association office in your state. Ask for the names and telephone numbers of programs near you.

To find a diabetes educator, call the American Association of Diabetes Educators, at 1-800-TEAM-UP-4 (800-832-6874). The operator will give you the names of several diabetes educators in your zip code.

To find an RD call 1-800-366-1655. This is the National Center for Nutrition and Dietetics at The American Dietetic Association. Ask for RDs in your area who specialize in diabetes and nutrition counseling.

Support is nearby

Nothing helps more than talking to someone who understands. You can often find support and lend an ear in a support group for people with diabetes. It's the place to gain valuable tips on better ways to manage your diabetes.

To find a support group

▲ Call 1-800-DIA-BETES (800-342-2383) to reach the American Diabetes Association office in your state. Ask about support groups in your area. Find out the focus of the group, the age range of the members, and when and where they meet.

▲ Call a nearby hospital to see whether they have a diabetes program.

▲ Call a local diabetes education program.

▲ Call the office of a local endocrinologist, diabetologist, or diabetes educator.

▲ Ask your pharmacist.

Good luck on your road to healthy eating, good diabetes control, and a long and healthy life!

INDEX